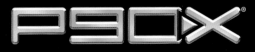

EXTREME TRAINING SYSTEM

FORGET

"I CAN'T"

AND SAY, **"I PRESENTLY STRUGGLE WITH."**

**A note from one of the first people to try the completed P90X® system,
Carl Daikeler, CEO of Beachbody® and Team Beachbody®:**

My, oh my . . . I just started week 2 of P90X, and in my personal frustration with feeling uncoordinated with much of the program, I spoke to Jon Congdon, President of Beachbody, about my "issues." He gave me a little insight into his first 30 days, since he was the VERY first to go through it: "I was sore the entire time, and Ab Ripper X was particularly challenging, grunting out 10, 15 reps on each move, max," he said. But by the end of 90 days, Jon was nailing it all.

EMBRACE THE STRUGGLE

The reason I'm going to beat the drum of "it's okay if you're struggling" is that I don't want you to quit if you struggle. I like to conquer stuff, and am generally surprised when I can't master something in one or two attempts. If you feel that way, you're not alone.

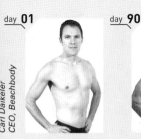

day **01**   day **90**

Carl Daikeler
CEO, Beachbody

I posted my progress on our Message Boards, logged in to WOWY®, our online SuperGym®, to work out with my crew, and participated in chats a couple of times a week. All along the way I met other people who were struggling, so I didn't feel quite as much like I was doing it all wrong or there was no hope for me. It was just that, a struggle. And struggle is where the growth is. Along with the folks on the boards and in WOWY, I kept it going for the full 90 days. The extreme results came with extreme commitment.

This is why you should seriously consider joining our online diet and support community at TeamBeachbody.com, where you'll find the ultimate tools and motivation you need to succeed. The Team Beachbody online diet and support club is where you can create your own personalized meal plan, take advantage of Tony's Corner—the place to go for VIP advice and live chats with the master of motivation himself—and get tips from your Coach.

And here's your ultimate motivation to "Bring It!®"—the Million Dollar Body Game®, which allows you to win up to $1,000 just for entering your workout in WOWY. Play daily so you don't miss it! Plus you can submit your Success Story every month for a chance to win cash and prizes and qualify for the $25,000 Grand Prize!

I so appreciate the enthusiasm the members of our community maintain throughout this intense and challenging program. And I'm proud to work hard to keep up with them. Now that you've decided to go for it, I truly hope you take advantage of these important tools like I did. You just need to log in, raise your hand, and say, "Who's in with me?"

Bring It!

Carl

_CARL DAIKELER
CEO, Beachbody and Team Beachbody

TABLE OF CONTENTS

Warning: Due to the physical nature of this program, Beachbody recommends that you get a complete physical examination from your physician before getting started.

TABLE OF CONTENTS

Record your rep count and weight amount on your FREE P90X Worksheets, downloadable at **P90XWorkoutSheets.com** or **TeamBeachbody.com/P90X**.

DO
YOUR
BEST
AND **FORGET THE REST.**

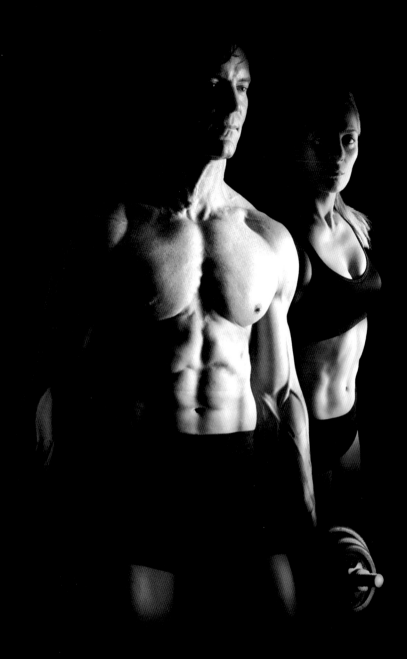

THIS IS P90X.

12 workout routines.

A 3-phase nutritional plan.

Premier training supplements.

And Tony Horton.

This is real training, and it starts by reading this book.

P90X SUCCESS STORIES

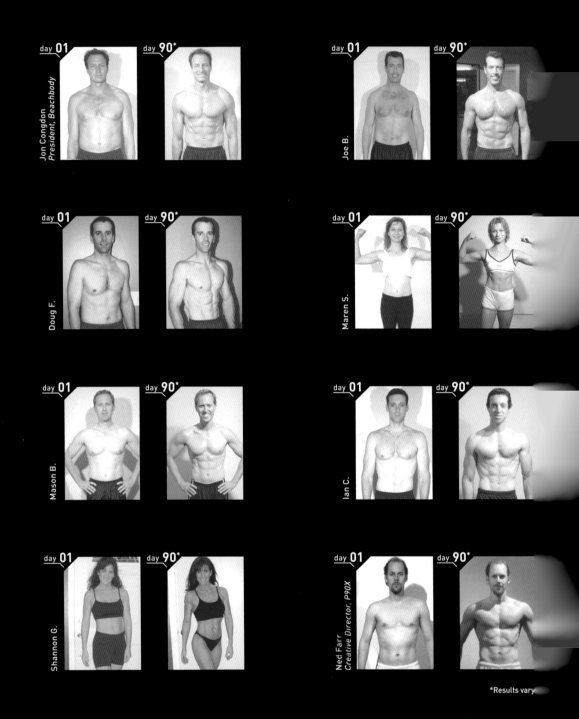

day 01 / day 90*

Jon Congdon
President, Beachbody

Joe B.

Doug F.

Maren S.

Mason B.

Ian C.

Shannon G.

Ned Farr
Creative Director, P90X

*Results vary

DO YOU REALLY HAVE TO READ

Unlike your DVD player manual, this guidebook is required reading. This is a vital tool that will outline your safest and most accurate path to succeed in this program. And you won't just be reading it; you'll be using it to give your journey direction and guidance every step of the way. (Just be sure to put it down when you're actually doing the exercises!)

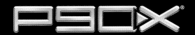

If you want to get totally ripped and get in the best shape of your life, this program is for you.

Even if you've already got the physical ability to participate, you'll still need to bring an extreme attitude and commitment to get to the P90X finish line.

WHO EXACTLY IS P90X FOR?

If you're unsure whether or not you're in good enough condition to take on this extreme fitness program, see the minimum suggested requirements in the Fit Test section of this guidebook. If you're unable to perform the minimum required reps for most of the exercises (or find the need to call the paramedics within minutes after popping in the first video), P90X may still be for you . . . but not just yet. In these cases, we would advise you to complete Beachbody's Power 90® or 10-Minute Trainer® before progressing to this advanced program. Finally, it's best to consult with your physician prior to beginning any exercise program, especially one as intense as P90X.

P90X is an extreme fitness program designed for individuals in top physical condition and health, and therefore should NOT be attempted by someone who doesn't meet the minimum fitness requirements outlined in this guidebook, or by someone who has any history of health problems, including but not limited to heart, respiratory, knee, shoulder, or spinal (back or neck) problems. This warning must not be discounted. There are many fitness alternatives if you have any physical or health conditions or are prone to injuries—but P90X is NOT one of them. The user assumes all risk of injury in the use of this program.

WHAT CAN YOU EXPECT?

To get in the best shape of your life.

To develop skills, coordination, and flexibility you never dreamed possible.

To sharpen your knowledge of smart eating and discover healthy diet choices.

And you can expect to sweat. A lot.

Just keep in mind that not all men and women are created equal. We come in a variety of shapes, sizes, and strengths, and therefore should have different expectations when it comes to results. P90X recognizes these differences and is designed to ensure that each individual is able to achieve his or her personal fitness goals. And that means YOU will achieve your goal.

From intense weight training to extreme yoga, you'll experience a variety of unique and challenging moves that will slim, strengthen, tone, and firm you and help you add muscle mass. We'll teach you how to control your results so you get what you want. With P90X, you can take your body where you want it to go.

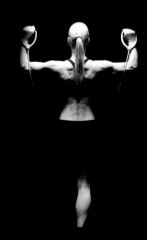

P90X is unlike any other exercise program ever devised. With a total of 12 separate workouts that contain hundreds of unique movements, this comprehensive fitness program will vault you to the next level and then some.

HOW DOES P90X GET YOU THERE?

Two words: **Muscle Confusion™.**

By providing an extensive variety of different moves that take time to master, P90X is continually challenging the body's muscles into new growth. The more you confuse the muscle, the harder your body has to work to keep up; the more variety you put into your workout, the better and faster your results will be.

The flaw with many fitness products is that they lead to a "plateau" where the body becomes accustomed to the routines, resulting in diminished effectiveness. P90X avoids this plateau effect **CONFUSED?** by switching things up to keep the body guessing for the entire 90 days. This means IT NEVER GETS EASY. By breaking old routines and opening new doors, secondary and tertiary (that's "thirdiary," but thirdiary isn't a word for some reason) muscles are constantly being activated and developed. P90X will continually challenge your body with its Muscle Confusion technique, utilizing what we call training "blocks."

KEEP READING

Each training block consists of 3 weeks of intensity, followed by 1 week of recovery. (Note: Don't think the term "recovery" means lying on a hammock all day sipping drinks with tiny umbrellas in them. The recovery week is defined in more detail later in this section.)

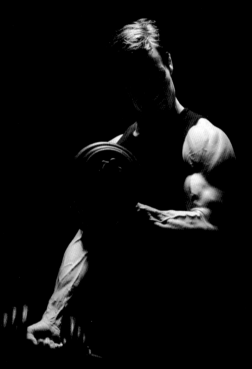

You will complete three training blocks in your 90 days, each building on gains made in the previous block. Nothing stays the same for long in this program. Routines are frequently switched, and aching muscles pay the price early on if you push yourself too hard. But for those animals able both to both pace their intensity and to hang in there and give it all they've got for 90 days as they get stronger, the payoff will be tremendous.

Within each training block there are also 3 phases: **1) The Adaptive phase**, when the body learns how to do the new set of exercises, followed by **2) the Mastery phase**, when the body responds to these exercises and experiences changes, and finally, **3) the Recovery phase**, when muscular healing occurs and your body grows strong, ready to be "confused" again.

Remember that your body only gets stronger while at rest, so the value of a well-designed recovery week—like the one in P90X—is essential to getting the most out of any exercise program. Don't let the name fool you; P90X's recovery week is no walk in the park. It'll probably challenge you as much as any other week in this program. However, it'll provide a break from heavy resistance training and will allow the microtrauma (small tears in the muscle) accumulated over the prior few weeks to heal so you can push even harder during the next training block.

**EXERCISE IS THE ARCHITECT.
RECOVERY IS THE BUILDER.**

"All well-organized training programs work in blocks to force your body to continually adapt to new exercise movements, cadences, or resistance. Increasing the speed, duration, or weight added to a given exercise is an obvious extension, and an important part of the process. But new movements are probably the most vital components of each block, as they are most challenging to the body."

Steve Edwards
Beachbody Fitness Advisor

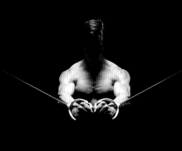

Any time you present your body with a new physical challenge, it must learn to develop a new set of "engrams," which are neuromuscular patterns developed in order to do the new movements. This learning process is referred to as an

YOU'LL ADAPT MORE QUICKLY, LEADING TO LONGER GROWTH PHASES

adaptive phase, which usually lasts 2 to 4 weeks, but may last as long as 10 weeks for untrained athletes. For this reason, more basic workout programs change your schedule less often. The more advanced the program, the shorter the training blocks, because a finely tuned body will adjust to new exercises much more quickly. P90X follows the "3 weeks on, 1 week off" pattern favored by athletes at the pinnacle of their sport.

The body always follows an adaptive phase with a dramatic growth phase. It then will naturally plateau as these movements become second nature. In P90X, we call the first block the adaptive phase. During the first month, your body will be in a state of neuromuscular confusion. Then, just when it feels it's getting things down, you'll switch again. In the successive blocks you'll adapt more quickly, leading to longer growth phases. This way, instead of hitting a plateau somewhere along the line, your growth curve will continue to climb skyward.

The following charts identify the dramatic difference between the traditional fitness program and P90X.

TRADITIONAL FITNESS PROGRAM

In a traditional fitness program, this sequence leads to a plateau.
See Figure_1 on next page

[1]_Adaptive and Mastery phase

[2]_Plateau (leveling off of growth)

WITH P90X

With P90X there is NO plateau. See Figure_2 on next page

[1]_Adaptive and Mastery phases

[4]_Recovery phase*

[2]_Recovery phase*

[5]_Adaptive and Mastery phases

[3]_Adaptive and Mastery phases

[6]_Recovery phase*

*Allows muscles to recover to peak strength, so you're ready for the intensity of the next adaptive phase.

With P90X you will:

_Use resistance for muscle tone and growth.**

_Execute isometric and dynamic body weight exercises for strength and power.

_Perform yoga, martial arts, gymnastics, and Pilates moves for coordination, balance, flexibility, core stabilization, and cardiovascular efficiency.

_Burn fat and expose your six-pack (maybe even your eight-pack!).

**When we say growth, we are NOT talking about bulk. We're talking about stamina and strength. However, if your top priority is to add some size to your physique, you can certainly achieve that with P90X as well.

By presenting so many complex and challenging movements, P90X forces you to continually adapt, ensuring new muscle growth and strength gains.

figure 1
TRADITIONAL PLATEAU EFFECT

MASTERY

ADAPTIVE

PLATEAU PLATEAU PLATEAU PLATEAU PLATEAU PLATEAU PLATEAU PLATEAU PLATEAU PLATEAU PLATEAU PLATEAU

PLATEAU PLATEAU PLATEAU PLATEAU PLATEAU PLATEAU PLATEAU PLATEAU PLATEAU PLATEAU PLATEAU PLATEAU

TIME

figure 2
ACCELERATED PROGRESS

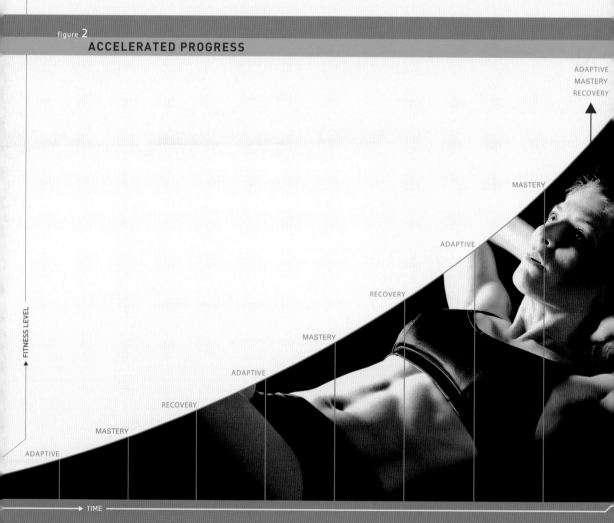

ADAPTIVE
MASTERY
RECOVERY

MASTERY

ADAPTIVE

RECOVERY

MASTERY

ADAPTIVE

RECOVERY

MASTERY

ADAPTIVE

FITNESS LEVEL

TIME

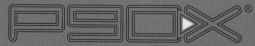

NUTRITION
aka, eat right, or why bother?

Just as this unique workout approach plays a vital role in maximizing your results, so does the food you choose to eat each day. Maintaining a healthy and nutritionally balanced diet designed to support extreme fitness is an integral part of this program. There is NO compromising in this area. By combining the right foods along with a sufficient amount of rest, P90X can propel you into the best shape of your life. If you keep eating junk, you'll still get fit—but you won't look it.

You'll find the P90X Nutrition Plan comprehensive yet surprisingly easy to follow, as you'll have plenty of delicious foods to choose from (although we can pretty much assure you none of them will have cream filling). P90X isn't about restricting calories or crash diets; it's about making the proper food choices to fuel your body for maximum performance. Did we mention there is NO compromising in this area?

We mean it.

A WORD FROM YOUR TRAINER, TONY HORTON

The food and snacks you put in your mouth will directly affect the quality of your life. Years of studies have shown that eating high-quality foods greatly reduces the risk and possibility of developing a variety of serious health problems. High-quality foods and supplements assist in lowering fat stores, losing weight, increasing energy, recovering from workouts, and maintaining healthy bones, muscles, and joints.

FOOD AS FUEL
Supplementation and eating well can also reduce feelings of depression, sadness, and anxiety while promoting psychological well-being.

The material in the P90X Nutrition Plan will show you what kinds of foods to eat and when to eat them. It will also explain why the supplements are a critical component for achieving maximum results. Showing up for six workouts each week requires discipline. It's also important to show restraint and discipline when it comes to your choices regarding food and supplementation. Your body doesn't run on exercise; it runs on the fuel you put in your mouth.

SUCCESS WITH P90X HINGES ON 3 THINGS:

*Variety_* This program provides plenty of that.

2 *Intensity_* Tony will show you how to focus on certain techniques that will help you reach "the Line" without going over it. Then it's up to you to Bring It!

3 *Consistency_* You must keep Pushing Play 6 days a week. Missing workouts, eating well only on occasion, and forgetting to take your supplements will adversely affect your energy, recovery, and results.

If you bring the same level of consistency and discipline to your daily fuel intake as you do to the workouts, you'll greatly reduce a lifetime of health risks, improve your overall quality of life, and see results from this program you never thought possible.

Tony Horton
Creator of the P90X Fitness Routines

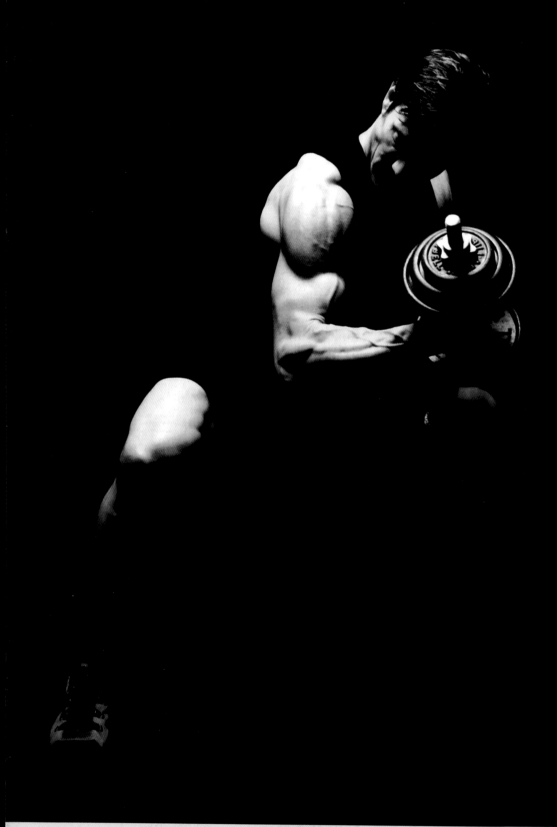

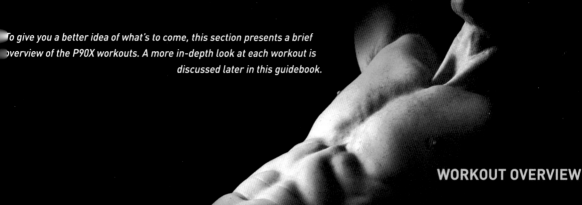

To give you a better idea of what's to come, this section presents a brief overview of the P90X workouts. A more in-depth look at each workout is discussed later in this guidebook.

WORKOUT OVERVIEW

01 CHEST & BACK
Workout Time _52:50

It's all about pushing and pulling during this resistance workout. With 12 dynamic exercises to strengthen, tighten, tone, and build the major muscles of the upper torso, you'll quickly feel the burn. While the majority of exercises will be either push-ups or pull-ups, there are a few that will require the use of dumbbells or bands.

02 PLYOMETRICS
Workout Time _58:36

You'd better Bring It! when you take on this dynamic cardio workout (some call it "the Beast"). With more than 30 explosive jumping moves, you won't be spending much time on the ground during this routine. Just be sure to wear some shock-absorbing footwear and work with a good shock-absorbing mat.

03 SHOULDERS & ARMS
Workout Time _59:53

Get out those dumbbells and/or bands. This workout incorporates a potent combination of pressing, curling, and fly movements that will do wonders for the development of the deltoid muscles (shoulders) and the biceps and triceps (arms).

04 YOGA X
Workout Time _92:24

If you think this'll be the day to relax and take a breather, forget it. This yoga workout will challenge you like never before. You'll sweat, twist, stretch, and hold all kinds of unfamiliar positions, but you'll leave feeling energized, invigorated, and maybe even a little enlightened.

05 LEGS & BACK
Workout Time _58:56

Get ready to squat, lunge, and pull during this unique series of exercises for both the lower and upper body. While the main focus lies in strengthening and developing the glutes, quads, hamstrings, and calves, there's also a handful of some highly effective pull-up exercises to give your legs a quick breather while you work the upper body. Some of the leg exercises during this routine require the use of dumbbells or bands.

06 KENPO X
Workout Time _55:46

The word Kenpo means "law of the fist," and that's exactly what you'll be throwing during this cardio-intense workout. That and a whole bunch of kicks, elbows, knees, and forearms. You'll learn a highly effective way to defend yourself, while at the same time getting one heck of a total-body, super-cardio workout.

07 X STRETCH
Workout Time _57:32

Keeping limber and loose is vital to the success of any fitness program. Aside from the stretching exercises that take place before, during, and after each P90X workout, we've created this entire 57-minute stretching routine to minimize the potential for injury and keep you at the top of your game.

08 CORE SYNERGISTICS
Workout Time _57:27

This total-body workout incorporates cardio, stretching, and resistance to strengthen the core muscles (the muscle groups that gird the waistline and back). Building a solid foundation with strong supporting muscles is the goal of this state-of-the-art workout. By strengthening your core, you'll be more prepared to tackle the resistance and cardio moves throughout this program, while reducing the chance of injury. You'll also improve your flexibility, balance, and coordination—all vital to the success of your total-body development.

09 CHEST, SHOULDERS & TRICEPS
Workout Time _55:44

You'll want to hit the beach and show off your lean, ripped muscles after finishing this intense upper-body blowout. This routine combines a variety of fun and challenging moves that will hit new muscles to build up your strength and definition. Push-ups, dips, flys, and tricep kickbacks constitute the majority of the exercises.

10 BACK & BICEPS
Workout Time _51:36

If Popeye had a favorite P90X workout, this would be it. With a boatload of curls and pull-ups, you'll add some real ammo to your guns. But don't worry, ladies—by using lighter weights, you can focus on toning and tightening those upper arms without adding the size that most guys are trying to develop. Additionally, this workout also provides some great definition to the back.

11 CARDIO X
Workout Time _43:18

In this workout, you'll keep your heart rate well below its anaerobic threshold, the point where strength gains are made and muscle fiber is broken down. Instead, you'll sweat comfortably as your body pumps oxygenated blood through your system, flushing out lactic acid and increasing your number of capillaries. This routine can be performed in addition to your standard P90X workload, or as a substitute if your body needs a break.

12 AB RIPPER X
Workout Time _16:07

This quick routine takes only 16 minutes to complete, yet still hits all areas of the midsection to burn the fat and tone the muscle. From sit-ups to Pilates moves, you'll find everything you need to flatten your stomach and get the six-pack you've always wanted.

ADDITIONAL EXTREME TRAINING WORKOUTS: P90X PLUS™

This is the next level of P90X extreme total-body training. Includes five intense new cardio, muscle-chiseling, and ab-/core-ripping moves to incorporate with P90X and get you ripped beyond belief.

P90X is an extremely intense fitness program. Sheer will and determination may get you to the finish line, but to achieve the best results, you've got to have the proper quality and quantity of nutrition. We make these supplements optional, so you have a choice. But know that P90X supplements were designed for this program and will supply your body with the nutrients necessary to give you added strength, energy, and stamina for each workout.

SUPPLEMENTS

WHY

THIS

PROGRAM

REALLY

REQUIRES

SUPPLEMENTS

Keep in mind, supplements are not drugs. A prescribed drug is taken when your body or mind is no longer capable of functioning normally. Supplements are taken to subtly assist the mind and body to naturally reach beyond normal everyday activities.

The cornerstone supplements identified below have been created to help you get the most from your efforts throughout this program.

Note: We don't trust a supplement that promises to do something for nothing. The P90X system is what we like to call "supplement assisted."

P90X SUPPLEMENTS

P90X® PEAK HEALTH FORMULA®

This formula is a complete multivitamin supplement (in capsule form) with added antioxidants, plant extracts, and other important phytonutrients, some of which are simply unobtainable in these amounts from a normal diet. This highly potent supplement contains more than 45 nutrients to supply comprehensive support for all areas of the body. Additionally, this formula provides anti-aging, anti-stress, cardiovascular, energy, immune system, and memory support. There is no other formula we know of with so many quality ingredients, in such high amounts, that covers as many bases. Taken daily, this unique blend of vitamins and minerals will keep you at the top of your game. Just like it does for Tony.*

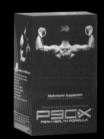

Recommended dosage: One packet of six per day, taken either all at once or divided between two or three meals . . . always with food.

P90X RESULTS AND RECOVERY FORMULA®

Extensive scientific research has shown that there is a 60-minute "window of opportunity" immediately following exercise when muscle cells are maximally primed to repair, rebuild, and adapt from a workout. This great-tasting formula was specially designed to provide the precise nutrients you'll need to achieve maximum results from your P90X workouts. Proper post-workout nutrition is a key factor in how quickly and completely your body will recover, adapt, and benefit from exercise. With 40 grams of carbs, 12 grams of protein, B vitamins, electrolytes, a host of minerals, and a dash of creatine per serving, no other recovery drink is better suited to maximize glycogen replenishment and muscle resynthesis. Don't be surprised if you find yourself working out just so you can drink this stuff.*

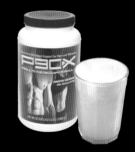

Recommended dosage: One serving (two scoops), preferably within an hour after your workout.

P90X® PEAK PERFORMANCE PROTEIN BARS

Unlike most other energy bars on the market today, these delicious protein bars pack 20 grams of protein each. Additionally, each bar contains no more than 7 grams of fat and no more than 270 calories. As an essential component for the growth and repair of muscle tissue, it's extremely beneficial to find healthy, great-tasting protein sources that can be consumed when a nutritious meal is unavailable.*

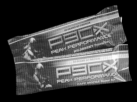

Recommended dosage: At least one bar a day as an alternative to a meal will naturally support your fat-loss goals while delivering healthy fuel to tone muscle.

For these and other great products, visit **P90XHome.com**, or if you're a member of the Team Beachbody community, contact your Coach or go to **TeamBeachbody.com/P90X**.

RECOVERY IS EVERYTHING

"When it comes to training, recovery is everything. The intense exercises in P90X require optimum recovery in order to get the most out of this extreme program. A good diet and proper rest will help to ensure that recovery, but science has discovered additional shortcuts you can use to speed up and further improve your recovery. Taking advantage of that science, we designed these P90X supplements specifically for maximizing your performance and recovery."

Mark Sisson
P90X Supplement Designer

Fitness and sports nutrition expert Mark Sisson has spent more than 20 years researching and designing state-of-the-art performance products and health-enhancing supplement products. His vast knowledge and experience in the fields of health, nutrition, and fitness have enabled him to create the perfect blend of supplements to safely and naturally enhance the results of your P90X workouts.

ADDITIONAL RECOMMENDED SUPPLEMENTS

Along with the P90X supplements, three additional supplements are highly recommended for optimal conditioning.

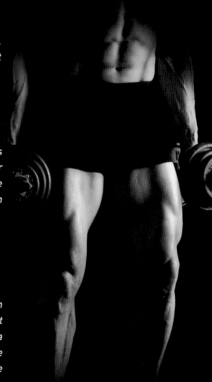

BEACHBODY
STRENGTH & MUSCLE MEN'S FORMULA

Up to four times more absorbable than regular creatine, our safe and potent formulation is a great-tasting way to get stronger and perform better.*

BEACHBODY
WHEY PROTEIN POWDER

With 18 grams of high-quality whey protein per serving, this is an easy way to ensure that you get enough protein in your diet to meet the rigorous demands of P90X. Additionally, the chocolate and vanilla flavors are among the best-tasting on the market. Grab a straw!

BEACHBODY
JOINT SUPPORT SUPER FORMULA

Our Super Formula combines glucosamine sulfate, collagen type II, and MSM in the proper ratios to be called the best joint support formula available today. Regular use of this formula can help keep your tendons and joints healthy and offset some of the effects of aging that are associated with degenerative bone and connective tissue problems. This product is especially recommended for those over the age of 40.*

The following equipment is recommended for use with P90X.

P90X JUMP MAT

With hundreds of exercise mats to choose from, only one had what it took to bring it to P90X. This high-quality, shock-absorbing mat will reduce the stress placed on your joints and tendons during the P90X Plyometrics workouts, and will provide a secure and comfortable surface for the Yoga X routines.

P90X CHIN-UP BAR

Pull-ups are an integral movement for upper-body development, and for this reason P90X requires a bar that can be used for a variety of pull-up exercises. Beachbody has designed the ultimate pull-up/chin-up bar to securely fit in most doorways. This valuable workout tool is ideal for performing the array of pull-up exercises used in this program.

DUMBBELLS

A major portion of P90X calls for weight resistance exercises to build strength and muscle. Depending on your fitness level, you will need a variety of dumbbells ranging in weight from 5 to 70 pounds.

B-LINES®
RESISTANCE BANDS

Some people prefer bands to dumbbells—especially if you travel. And results can be even more dramatic when you use bands. Beachbody offers bands with ergonomic handles for maximum comfort during even the most intense movements. For men we recommend a three-band kit that includes Magenta (B4), Red (B6), and Green (B8). For women we recommend a three-band kit that includes Pink (B3), Magenta (B4), and Red (B6).

HEART RATE MONITOR

Gauge the intensity level and calorie burn from your workout with Beachbody's reliable and easy-to-use heart rate monitor. A must for all those taking their fitness regimen to the next level.

YOGA BLOCKS (2)

For those new to yoga and the slightly less flexible, these blocks offer added support to assist with balance while holding certain poses.

BODY FAT TESTER

Getting an accurate reading of your body fat percentage will allow you to clearly identify and measure your fat-loss accomplishments throughout this program.

TONY HORTON'S
POWERSTANDS®

If your chest is already strong enough to knock out three sets of 20-plus push-ups each, these non-skid push-up stands designed by Tony Horton are the ideal tool for intensifying your movements. They can also be a benefit to those who suffer from wrist ailments, as the unique ergonomic design helps alleviate stress on the wrist joints.

SELECTTECH® DUMBBELLS

They provide a revolutionary new way to lift weights—you can build fat-burning muscle with the turn of a dial. These space-saving dumbbells give you all the weights you need in just one set!

For these and other great products, visit **P90XHome.com**, or if you're a member of the Team Beachbody community, contact your Coach or go to **TeamBeachbody.com/P90X**.

LESSENING YOUR CHANCE OF INJURY

During any training program, you're at risk of getting injured. For this reason you should always err on the side of caution when exercising. P90X is going to be hard for everyone at some point. It's too varied not to take you out of your comfort zone, no matter how seasoned an athlete you are. But you can stack the odds in your favor by training smart, and following a few simple rules.

EXERCISE ON THE SIDE OF CAUTION.

Don't cross the threshold.

The fact is that the harder you train, the closer you come to the threshold where you could become injured should you cross it. Realizing that this point exists is rule number one. You have a limit! Look out for it. Respect it.

Stay in control.

There are times to push as hard as you can, but you've got to draw the line somewhere. Back off once your muscles really start to shake. At this point, you're likely to lose your ability to maintain proper form.

Maintain proper form.

Never compromise form in order to finish a set. When the muscles you're working give out, it's time to stop. Don't try to engage other muscles just to finish. It's not worth it. Part of the goal of P90X is to complement the natural "blueprint" of your body. So check your form, and work out in a way that's kind to your structure. That'll keep you healthy while you get strong.

Warm up.

If you don't feel sufficiently warm (your body should feel limber and break a light sweat), hit pause and warm up some more. You can't over-warm up, but you can certainly under-warm up. Never let the way someone else feels cloud your judgment.

Listen to your body.

No one knows better than you do: If something feels wrong, it probably is. Learn to stop at any discomfort. Then assess the situation and decide whether it's a physical problem or whether you're just having an off day. This isn't a race. If you stay healthy, results will come plenty fast. If you push too hard, you can get hurt, and—BAM!—you're on the sideline. The goal is to complete this program. Don't try to peak on day 2.

As with any difficult challenge, it can be a tremendous advantage to have support from others who are going through the same program. When times are tough during P90X, having friends and family members to cheer you on every step of the way can make all the difference in getting you to the finish line.

SUPPORT

CHEER YOU ON!

BEACHBODY® MESSAGE BOARDS

Additional support during your P90X journey can also be found on the Message Boards. Just visit Beachbody.com/P90X, or if you're a member of the Team Beachbody community, go to TeamBeachbody.com. While at first it may seem awkward to share your thoughts, concerns, and questions with total strangers, you'll quickly discover how helpful and totally cool these people really are. No matter how busy, tired, or sore you may be, on the boards you'll find some sympathetic soul experiencing the same highs and lows as you. This type of team support will give you the encouragement to persevere to the end, and it's available to anyone with access to the Internet. Once you start to see the kind of amped-up excitement people are talking about in the P90X forum, you'll be hooked. Seeing the remarkable strides made by others has proven to be a highly successful motivating force. You'll most likely find yourself saying, "If that guy/gal can do it, I sure as hell/heck can too."

In fact, now you can even schedule workouts with other P90Xers around the country—just log on to WOWY, Beachbody's online SuperGym, and make an appointment to Push Play. By arranging to "meet" online at a specific time with others who are experiencing similar P90X trials and tribulations, you'll be much more likely to stick with the program. Plus, each time you enter your workout, you'll qualify for the daily prize of up to $1,000! With WOWY, you're never alone!

TEAM BEACHBODY® ONLINE DIET AND SUPPORT CLUB

At the Team Beachbody online diet and support club, you'll get an expanded package of personalized weight loss and fitness support tools to help ensure the best possible results throughout this intense program. Team Beachbody is a vital resource and it's there for you! Online you'll get:

Live Access to Tony Horton_ Tell the man who brings you to the brink of total exhaustion each day what's on your mind, and hear his entertaining words of inspiration.

Your Personalized Meal Plans_ An interactive tool to create easy-to-follow meal plans customized just for you! We'll show you the right foods to eat in the right portions, so there's no guesswork.

Interactive Diet and Fitness Tools_ Monitor your progress in your P90X journey with effective, easy-to-use online tools proven to help you succeed.

Expert Advice_ Our highly qualified fitness advisors and our team of experts provide thorough answers to help you choose the right mix of foods and supplements to fuel your workout, and perform each exercise correctly to minimize the risk of injury. You'll also be able to choose a personal Coach who'll keep you informed and motivated every step of the way.

P90X Success_ Whether it's Tony Horton, a Team Beachbody Coach, a team of virtual workout partners, or state-of-the art diet and fitness tools, you'll find all the support you need to maintain your intensity for the full 90 days. Take advantage of Team Beachbody to get the most out of your daily efforts and achieve real and lasting P90X success.

Extraordinary Prizes_ Play the Million Dollar Body Game® and you can win prizes for submitting your Success Story. Plus when you work out in WOWY, our online SuperGym, you are automatically entered to win our daily prize!

_ARMS

_BICEPS The bicep comprises 40 percent of the upper arm. The main function of the bicep is to move the forearm toward the shoulder (elbow flexion). The secondary function of the bicep is to rotate the wrist.

_TRICEPS The triceps muscle is composed of three separate heads. Together they make up 60 percent of the upper-arm muscle mass. The main function of the triceps is to straighten the arm and bring it down toward the body.

_BACK

_LATS (latissimus dorsi) are the large muscles on either side of the back. Their primary function is to pull the arm down from overhead. When the arm is stable, the lats act to lift the body up toward the shoulders. The lats also help stabilize the torso during many pressing movements.

_TRAPS (trapezius) are long, trapezoid-shaped muscles that run down the upper portion of the spine. Bringing the shoulder blades together, pulling the shoulder blades down, and shrugging the shoulders up are the main functions of these muscles.

_CHEST

_PECS (pectorals) These muscles attach near the shoulder joint and originate on the breastbone in the center of the chest. The fibers of these muscles run across the entire chest region. The pecs serve to bring the arm across the chest and to move it forward in the shoulder socket.

_LEGS

_CALVES The calf muscle originates behind the knee and attaches to the heel with the Achilles tendon. Its primary function is to raise the heel off the ground.

_GLUTES (gluteus maximus) These muscles originate along the pelvic bone and attach to the back of the upper leg. Extending the hip is their primary function.

_HAMSTRINGS These muscles originate just underneath the glutes. Their primary function is to bring the heel toward the buttocks and to move the leg to the rear.

_QUADS (quadriceps) Located on the front of the thigh, the main function of these powerful muscles is to support the upper body during a squatting movement.

_SHOULDERS

_DELTS (deltoids) Composed of three muscles (anterior, lateral, and posterior heads), the delts provide total mobility to the shoulder joint in all directions. These muscles play a vital role in the majority of upper-body exercises, including chest and shoulder presses. The main function of the deltoid is to move the arm away from the body.

_STOMACH

_ABS (abdominal muscles) This muscle group consists of:
  _ The rectus abdominus (the visible portion of the abs), which brings the rib cage toward the pelvis.
  _ The obliques (muscles at the waist), which rotate the torso and stabilize the abdomen.
  _ The transverse abdominus (muscle that supports the spine), which stabilizes the torso.

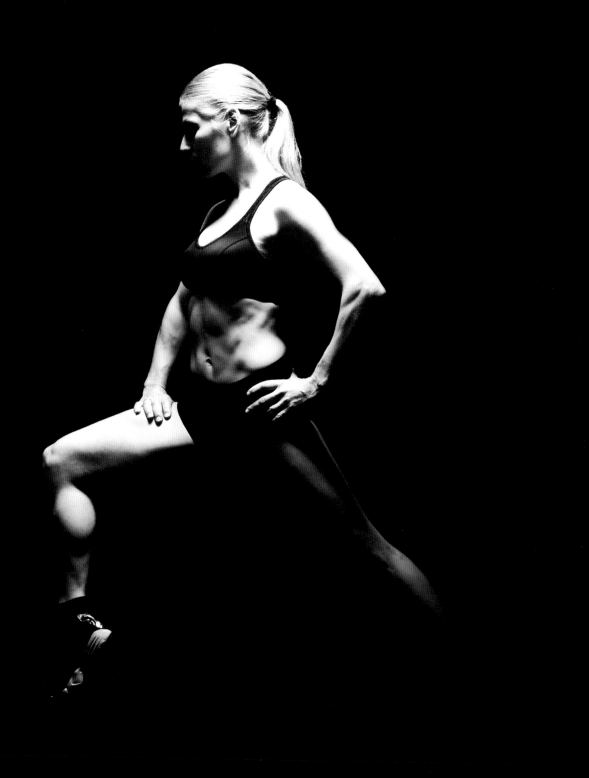

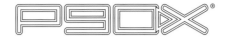

P90X PREP
things to do before you start the program

Step 1_Watch the *How to Bring It!* video.

Step 2_Record your measurements and take "before" photos.

Step 3_Take the Fit Test—are you ready for P90X?

Step 4_Get your kitchen in order (see the P90X Nutrition Plan).

Step 5_Visit **P90XWorkoutSheets.com** or **TeamBeachbody.com/P90X** to download your FREE P90X Worksheets and link to the P90X Message Boards for amazing support.

"BEFORE" AND "AFTER" BODY MEASUREMENTS

Since P90X increases muscle, and muscle weighs more than fat, you'll want to compare your body fat before and after for accurate body transformation results. Record your measurement data in the spaces provided below, as well as on page 4 of the P90X Nutrition Plan. If you're a member of the Team Beachbody community, go to TeamBeachbody.com to log your measurements.

BODY FAT %   Prior to Day 1 _____   After Day 90 _____ (also enter on page 3 of diet guide)

Use Beachbody's body fat tester to record your current body fat measurements. To get the most accurate readings, follow the directions on the package.

WEIGHT   Prior to Day 1 _____   After Day 90 _____ (please indicate if wearing any clothes)

CHEST   Prior to Day 1 _____"   After Day 90 _____"

WAIST   Prior to Day 1 _____"   After Day 90 _____"

HIPS   Prior to Day 1 _____"   After Day 90 _____"

RIGHT THIGH   Prior to Day 1 _____"   After Day 90 _____" (measured at midpoint)

LEFT THIGH   Prior to Day 1 _____"   After Day 90 _____" (measured at midpoint)

RIGHT ARM   Prior to Day 1 _____"   After Day 90 _____" (flexed, measured at peak of bicep)

LEFT ARM   Prior to Day 1 _____"   After Day 90 _____" (flexed, measured at peak of bicep)

"BEFORE" AND "AFTER" PHOTOS The more you show, the more you'll know. Wear a swimsuit, underwear, or something comparable so you can see where you need the work, and where you're making progress. Don't be afraid to show some skin. These photos are great motivators. Be sure to take your first series of photos prior to day 1, following these simple guidelines:

1. Use a plain background if possible.

2. Take a few front shots (hands on hips, "biceps flex" muscle pose), a few side shots (hands at sides), and a few back shots (hands on hips, "biceps flex" muscle pose).

3. Don't "suck it in" or "push it out." You want a true reflection of your body's appearance. This isn't just a "before" photo, it's a "goodbye" photo. The P90X train is about to leave the station, and that body is going to leave some luggage behind. "Whoo-whooo!"

4. Repeat this process after Phase 1, after Phase 2, and after Phase 3 to chart your visual progress.

5. Visit **P90XHome.com**, or if you're a member of the Team Beachbody community, go to **TeamBeachbody.com**, to create a profile page and post your photos online.

TAKE THE FIT TEST Before starting an extreme fitness program like P90X, it's important to know where you stand and if your current fitness level is adequate. Providing an honest assessment of your abilities and your mindset will allow you to take advantage of your strengths and overcome your weaknesses.

We ask that you complete the equivalent of Power 90® or Slim in 6® before you begin. But if you're unfamiliar with these programs, we've set some guidelines for you to follow. If you can't do what's listed on the following pages, you'll see better results if you do another exercise program before you take on P90X. So if you can't finish the Fit Test, do Power 90. You'll get great results, then be able to come back and crush P90X.

IMPORTANT NOTE Do this test a few days before your official "day 1." The P90X Fit Test takes approximately 40 minutes to complete. Be sure to perform all the exercises consecutively, in the order they appear. Keep up with the timing, and make a note if you do anything differently; you'll repeat this Fit Test when you complete P90X, so it is vital that you're able to do it the same way, in the same order. That way you'll get a true indication of the improvements you've made. Pay attention, and be honest with yourself.

WHAT YOU'LL NEED
TO TAKE THE FIT TEST

_Heart rate monitor
_Body fat tester or caliper
_Tape measure
_Scale (calibrate to 0.0 lbs.)
_Partner to help record data (optional)

_Chin-up bar (securely installed)
_Timer (stopwatch or watch with second hand)
_Towel
_Water
_Your "Bring It!" game face

THE FIT TEST
resting heart rate

You'll want to monitor your morning resting heart rate throughout this program. This is a good indicator of your overall cardiovascular fitness. If possible, take your resting heart rate as soon as you wake up (BEFORE GETTING OUT OF BED). Over the course of the program, your resting heart rate should drop. If it goes up a few days in a row, you may be overtraining or getting sick.

HOW TO TAKE YOUR RESTING HEART RATE

Put on your heart rate monitor. Be sure it's secure and working correctly before beginning. Try to be as relaxed as possible when taking this reading. Remain calm and quiet for 2 minutes, then record your resting heart rate below.

If you don't have a heart rate monitor, take your pulse from either your neck or wrist, and count the beats for 30 seconds. Multiply by two to get your resting heart rate.

Heart rate before **DAY 1:** _____

Heart rate after **DAY 90:** _____

That was the easy part . . . most likely you passed that.

NOW WARM UP:

Now take about 10 minutes to warm up. Start by marching in place, then do any low-impact movements you like (jumping jacks, light jog in place, etc.) until you build up a light sweat, then stretch out lightly. You never want to work "to failure" when you're cold and tight. The warm-up on Power 90 Cardio 3-4 through the yoga moves is a good way to get you ready.

1_PULL-UPS

maximum number of pull-ups to failure

Using wide grip, grasp your chin-up bar (palms facing forward, away from body, two fists wider than shoulders). From a hanging position, pull body up smoothly until chin clears the bar. Lower body back down, being sure to straighten your arms, and repeat without bouncing up. Don't be discouraged if you aren't able to do very many. Do as many as you can, to "failure."*

Record the number of pull-ups you can do here. (If you're only able to do 1/4, 1/2, or 3/4 of a pull-up, go ahead and record it anyway.)

*TO FAILURE?
Physically "to failure" is when your body stops you by not being able to go any further without causing injury. Do not force past failure.

Before **DAY 1:** _____

After **DAY 90:** _____

P90X Minimum_ Should be able to do at least 3 pull-ups if male, 1 pull-up if female. However, many people won't be able to do any pull-ups when starting P90X. You'll get more out of the program if you can do pull-ups, but you can substitute by using the B-LINES® Resistance Bands with the door attachment for pull-downs, which are demonstrated as an alternative in the videos.

REST 1 MINUTE BEFORE GOING ON TO THE NEXT EXERCISE.

2_VERTICAL LEAP

Stand sideways with shoulder against wall and raise arm straight overhead against the wall. Record that height here.

Before **DAY 1:** _____

After **DAY 90:** _____

jump with step

Then lower arm, take JUST ONE STEP back and proceed to jump straight up, trying to touch highest point on wall (no gathering up a head of steam prior to your jump—think "jump ball"). Record that height here.

Before **DAY 1:** _____

After **DAY 90:** _____

Subtract the first measurement from the second; that is your vertical leap. Record your vertical leap inches here.

Before **DAY 1:** _____

After **DAY 90:** _____

P90X Minimum_ **Should have a vertical leap of at least 5 inches if male, 3 inches if female.**

REST 4 MINUTES BEFORE GOING ON TO THE NEXT EXERCISE.

3_PUSH-UPS

maximum number of push-ups to failure

Put down something soft, about 2 or 3 inches high (pillow or cushion), to make contact with chest on each rep. Be sure to keep body straight with hands at "normal" push-up width.

Record number of push-ups performed to failure here.

Before **DAY 1:** _____

After **DAY 90:** _____

P90X Minimum_ **Should be able to do at least 15 if male, 3 if female (or 15 push-ups off your knees).**

REST 4 MINUTES BEFORE GOING ON TO THE NEXT EXERCISE.

4_TOE TOUCH

flexibility test

You will need a ruler or tape measure for this test. Sit on floor with legs extended directly in front of you. Bend forward at waist and extend arms over legs toward toes. Don't bend knees. See how close you can get fingertips to toes. If not able to reach, measure the distance from fingertips to toes. If able to extend fingers beyond toes, measure how much further fingers reach beyond toes. Do not strain or force.

Record distance from fingertips to toes here.

Use a "–" if not able to reach toes (e.g., –3 inches)
or a "+" if reaching beyond toes (e.g., +3 inches).

Before **DAY 1:**

After **DAY 90:**

P90X Minimum_   **Reach should be no less than 6 inches from your toes, or a "–6."**

REST 4 MINUTES BEFORE GOING ON TO THE NEXT EXERCISE.

5_WALL SQUAT

isolating quad/
leg strength

Place back flat against wall and lower your body into a seated chair position (quads parallel to the floor, feet directly below knees (think 90-degree angle here). Start timer as soon as you get into the chair position. Breathe through the discomfort and hang in there until you can't hold yourself up any longer (i.e., to failure). Be sure NOT to place hands on wall or "scoot" with shoulders. You can slide down slowly as you get tired, but once your butt touches the floor, time's up.

Record exact time able to hold wall squat here.

Before **DAY 1:**

After **DAY 90:**

P90X Minimum_   **Should be able to hold wall squat for at least 1 minute.**

REST 4 MINUTES BEFORE GOING ON TO THE NEXT EXERCISE.

Choice of weight is important for this exercise. A somewhat heavier weight will be more effective in helping you determine your results on day 90—think of the weight at which you will max out at 10 to15 reps. Men should consider a minimum of 20 pounds; women should consider a minimum of 8 pounds. (See minimum below.)

6_BICEP CURLS

front-facing curls

Extend arms straight down in front of body, palms forward. Be sure that arms are fully extended between each curl. Using both arms at the same time, perform as many curls as you can until failure. Don't rock or cheat, and no breaks longer than 1 second between reps.

Record number of curls completed and weight used here.

Before **DAY 1:**   number   weight

After **DAY 90:**   number   weight

P90X Minimum_   **Should be able to do at least 10 curls with 20 pounds. if male; at least 10 curls with 8 pounds. if female.**

REST 3 MINUTES BEFORE GOING ON TO THE NEXT EXERCISE.

7_IN AND OUTS

the ab test

Starting position: Seated with hands on the floor at your sides, knees bent with feet on the floor. Raise feet off the ground and bring knees in toward your chest. Straighten legs back out and repeat movement without touching floor.

Record number of in and outs performed here.

Before **DAY 1:**

After **DAY 90:**

P90X Minimum_   **Should be able to do at least 25.**

REST 4 MINUTES BEFORE GOING ON TO THE NEXT EXERCISE.

8_HEART RATE MAXIMIZER

You'll now perform jumping jacks nonstop for 2 minutes at a quick and steady pace. During the final 30 seconds, you'll go as fast as you can to maximize your heart rate. When you finish, be prepared to measure your heart rate over a span of 4 minutes. Should be able to finish the test standing and still able to breathe.

Step 1: Two minutes at quick and steady pace—last 30 seconds are at sprint.
Step 2: Record heart rate <u>immediately after</u> jumping jacks here.

Before **DAY 1:** _____

After **DAY 90:** _____

Step 3: Heart rate 1 minute from stopping here.

Before **DAY 1:** _____

After **DAY 90:** _____

Step 4: Heart rate 2 minutes from stopping here.

Before **DAY 1:** _____

After **DAY 90:** _____

Step 5: Heart rate 3 minutes from stopping here.

Before **DAY 1:** _____

After **DAY 90:** _____

Step 6: Heart rate 4 minutes from stopping here.

Before **DAY 1:** _____

After **DAY 90:** _____

P90X Minimum_   **Be able to finish the 2 minutes of jumping jacks.**

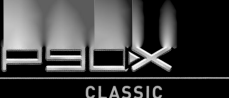

CLASSIC

IF YOU PASS ALL THE P90X MINIMUMS, TIME TO START

Consider this the starting line for the extreme physical and mental challenge ahead. It's time to show what you've got. It may take some time to get used to the rigors of this program, but with patience and determination, you'll go the distance.

P90X—BRING IT!

WEEKS 1–3

During this phase, your goal should be to master each movement and finish the workouts in one piece. So for now, focus less on the amount of weight you're lifting and instead try to achieve your desired number of repetitions while maintaining strict form. Remember to record your rep count and weight amount on your FREE P90X Worksheets, downloadable at **P90XWorkoutSheets.com** or **TeamBeachbody.com/P90X**.

PHASE 1

DAY_1 Chest & Back, Ab Ripper X

_2 Plyometrics

_3 Shoulders & Arms, Ab Ripper X

_4 Yoga X

_5 Legs & Back, Ab Ripper X

_6 Kenpo X

_7 Rest or X Stretch

RECOVERY AND AB FOCUS

After 3 weeks of taking a pounding, your body will be begging for some relief—and this transition comes just in time. Don't expect this week to be easy. As a matter of fact, it may seem harder than the previous weeks if cardiovascular fitness is your weak area. But it will allow your body to recover from the hard resistance training and will enhance your adaptive process. You'll also focus on tightening the entire midsection into a hard, ripped sheet. Core strength, balance, and flexibility are the focus of the week as your body increases its stabilizer-muscle strength during recovery and ab focus.

WEEK 4

DAY_1 Yoga X

_2 Core Synergistics

_3 Kenpo X

_4 X Stretch

_5 Core Synergistics

_6 Yoga X

_7 Rest or X Stretch

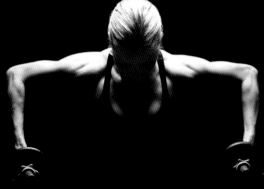

2

If you really want to add some size, now's the time to go for it. Use enough weight on each exercise so you max out at 8 to 10 reps. If you just want to continue developing lean muscle, use enough weight so you max out between 12 and 15 reps. Never do 11 . . . (we kid you). Also keep in mind that your body only builds muscle while at rest. So try to get at least 7 hours of sleep—which should be easy, because this schedule will wipe you out.

WEEKS 5-7

DAY_1 Chest, Shoulders & Triceps, Ab Ripper X

_2 Plyometrics

_3 Back & Biceps, Ab Ripper X

_4 Yoga X

_5 Legs & Back, Ab Ripper X

_6 Kenpo X

_7 Rest or X Stretch

RECOVERY AND AB FOCUS Once again, your body will thank you for a reprieve from the previous 3 weeks. This second recovery week brings back the workouts that focus on those seldom-used muscles, including the entire midsection. At this point you should be more comfortable performing the core exercises, and by the end of the week you'll begin to feel stronger and ready to hit the weights in the next phase.

WEEK 8

DAY_1 Yoga X

_2 Core Synergistics

_3 Kenpo X

_4 X Stretch

_5 Core Synergistics

_6 Yoga X

_7 Rest or X Stretch

Extreme Muscle Confusion is what this phase is all about. At the onset of this stage, you should be rested and ready to leave everything you've got on your exercise mat. No holding back. This will be the time to push to exhaustion and near muscle failure on every single set. Give it your maximum effort, each and every day, and you'll know the true meaning of X. C'mon—we dare you.

WEEKS 9 AND 11

DAY_1 Chest & Back, Ab Ripper X
_2 Plyometrics
_3 Shoulders & Arms, Ab Ripper X
_4 Yoga X
_5 Legs & Back, Ab Ripper X
_6 Kenpo X
_7 Rest or X Stretch

WEEKS 10 AND 12

DAY_1 Chest, Shoulders & Triceps, Ab Ripper X
_2 Plyometrics
_3 Back & Biceps, Ab Ripper X
_4 Yoga X
_5 Legs & Back, Ab Ripper X
_6 Kenpo X
_7 Rest or X Stretch

WEEK 13

DAY_1 Yoga X
_2 Core Synergistics
_3 Kenpo X
_4 X Stretch
_5 Core Synergistics
_6 Yoga X
_7 Rest or X Stretch

THE FINAL STRETCH By this point you should be in the best shape of your life, but it's not the time to prove it yet. Remember, strength improves and muscles grow while at rest. One more recovery week will get you into optimal condition to take your final Fit Test and "after" photos. And should you continue to move forward in your P90X training, this recovery week is a must.

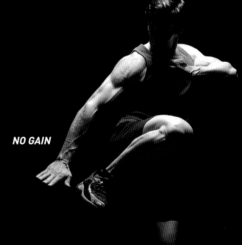

NO PAIN Often you'll hear the expression "No pain, no gain" when it comes to achieving fitness results. Understand that this doesn't refer to the kind of pain a trapeze artist would experience after missing the net. What it does refer to is muscle burn that's common during intense workouts. It's a GOOD pain. Let's review: missing-the-net pain, bad; muscle-burning pain during intense exercise, good!

NO GAIN

CAN YOU EXTEND EACH PHASE?

Given your newfound knowledge about the adaptive phase, this is an understandable question and a valid one. There are a few reasons why you may want to extend one or more phases of the program. Perhaps you had trouble learning the movements, had an "off" week when you didn't feel you pushed hard, got sick, or were just plain busy. It can be effective to continue a phase for an extended week or two, no problem. But never do a phase longer than 6 weeks. You'll always get better results by shaking things up on a regular basis.

Confused? Good, you're getting it—or at least your muscles are.

OTHER WAYS TO USE THE P90X ROUTINES

We offer two alternatives to the classic P90X routine. While both of these programs are designed to generate slightly different results, they're just as intense as the classic version. Additionally, they're good options for subsequent rounds of P90X. Just be sure to take at least a couple of weeks off between programs.

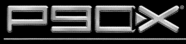

DOUBLES

The Doubles plan of attack is for those who want some extra cardiovascular exercise, either for performance or weight loss. Keep in mind that P90X is stressful within the realm of its standard schedule. Those attempting Doubles should be completely injury-free and have plenty of energy to add another workout to the schedule 3 or 4 days per week. The Cardio X workout is the least intense of the P90X series, but it's still a serious calorie-burner.

PHASE 1

This phase is identical to the classic way of doing P90X. During this phase your body will be adapting, and no further breakdown is likely to be beneficial. Remember to record your rep count and weight amount on your FREE P90X Worksheets, downloadable at **P90XWorkoutSheets.com** or **TeamBeachbody.com/P90X**.

WEEKS 1–3

DAY_1 Chest & Back, Ab Ripper X
_2 Plyometrics
_3 Shoulders & Arms, Ab Ripper X
_4 Yoga X
_5 Legs & Back, Ab Ripper X
_6 Kenpo X
_7 Rest or X Stretch

WEEK 4

DAY_1 Yoga X
_2 Core Synergistics
_3 Kenpo X *RECOVERY AND AB FOCUS*
_4 X Stretch
_5 Core Synergistics
_6 Yoga X
_7 Rest or X Stretch

PHASE 2

Here we go. Add Cardio X three times per week. It's recommended to do this workout in the morning on an empty stomach. Then do your regular P90X workout later when you've got more blood glycogen for energy.

WEEKS 5–7

DAY_1 AM Cardio X
PM Chest, Shoulders & Triceps, Ab Ripper X
_2 Plyometrics
_3 AM Cardio X
PM Back & Biceps, Ab Ripper X
_4 Yoga X
_5 AM Cardio X
PM Legs & Back, Ab Ripper X
_6 Kenpo X
_7 Rest or X Stretch

WEEK 8

DAY_1 Yoga X
_2 Core Synergistics
_3 Kenpo X *RECOVERY AND AB FOCUS*
_4 X Stretch
_5 Core Synergistics
_6 Yoga X
_7 Rest or X Stretch

With 4 days per week of cardio in addition to your regular schedule, you're going to have to eat very well to sustain the final 4 weeks. This is essentially "hell week," just like high school football season, except it's not 1 week, it's 4.

Note: If you start to feel excessively tired, don't be afraid to skip your morning workout. If you're overtraining, it's no longer beneficial, so pay close attention to your body and how it's reacting.

3 PHASE

WEEKS 9 AND 11

DAY_1 AM Cardio X
    PM Chest & Back, Ab Ripper X
_2 AM Cardio X
    PM Plyometrics
_3 Shoulders & Arms, Ab Ripper X
_4 AM Cardio X
    PM Yoga X
_5 AM Cardio X
    PM Legs & Back, Ab Ripper X
_6 Kenpo X
_7 Rest or X Stretch

WEEKS 10 AND 12

DAY_1 AM Cardio X
    PM Chest, Shoulders & Triceps, Ab Ripper X
_2 AM Cardio X
    PM Plyometrics
_3 Back & Biceps, Ab Ripper X
_4 AM Cardio X
    PM Yoga X
_5 AM Cardio X
    PM Legs & Back, Ab Ripper X
_6 Kenpo X
_7 Rest or X Stretch

WEEK 13

RECOVERY AND AB FOCUS

DAY_1 Yoga X
_2 Core Synergistics
_3 Kenpo X
_4 X Stretch
_5 Core Synergistics
_6 Yoga X
_7 Rest or X Stretch

WHEW—YOU'VE EARNED THIS WEEK!

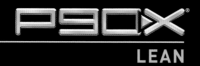

LEAN

**MORE CARDIO AND LESS RESISTANCE
FOR MAXIMUM WEIGHT LOSS**

P90X Lean is for those who want a more cardio-based and slightly less intensive program. Make no mistake, this is the real deal and no picnic. In fact, you may sweat more than in regular P90X. And what you sacrifice in overall gains in strength and speed, you'll make up for with positive changes in lean body mass.

During this period, your body's going to get accustomed to the rigors and demands of P90X by forming engrams, or neuromuscular patterns that allow you to turn new movements into routine. Your aim should be to finish each workout and perfect each movement, as opposed to focusing on weight or resistance. As your body gets used to the exercises, it will do them more efficiently, and the amount of weight you can use will greatly increase. You should begin to see this efficiency skyrocket toward the end of week 3. Remember to record your rep count and weight amount on your FREE P90X Worksheets, downloadable at **P90XWorkoutSheets.com** or **TeamBeachbody.com/P90X.**

WEEKS 1–3

PHASE 1

DAY_1 Core Synergistics
_2 Cardio X
_3 Shoulders & Arms, Ab Ripper X
_4 Yoga X
_5 Legs & Back, Ab Ripper X
_6 Kenpo X
_7 Rest or X Stretch

Before you get comfortable, you'll need to back off a bit. While it's not easy, this week will allow your body to recover from hard resistance training while continuing your adaptive process. Core strength, cardio, and flexibility are the focus of the week as your body builds more engrams and increases stabilizer-muscle strength.

WEEK 4

DAY_1 Yoga X
_2 Core Synergistics
_3 Kenpo X
_4 X Stretch
_5 Cardio X
_6 Yoga X
_7 Rest or X Stretch

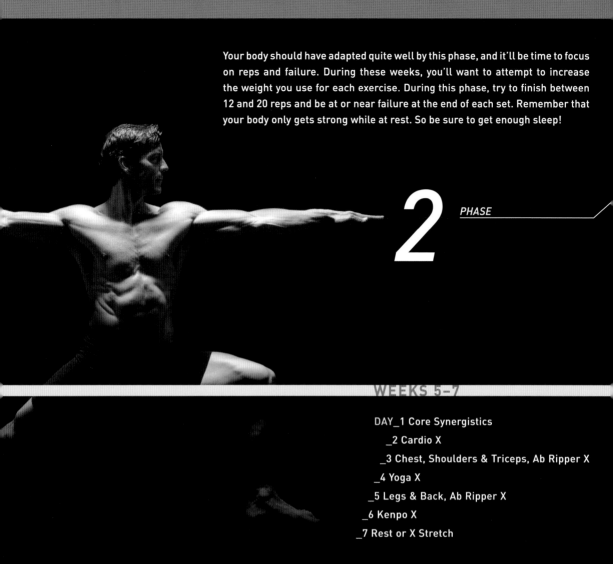

Your body should have adapted quite well by this phase, and it'll be time to focus on reps and failure. During these weeks, you'll want to attempt to increase the weight you use for each exercise. During this phase, try to finish between 12 and 20 reps and be at or near failure at the end of each set. Remember that your body only gets strong while at rest. So be sure to get enough sleep!

2 *PHASE*

WEEKS 5-7

DAY_1 Core Synergistics
   _2 Cardio X
   _3 Chest, Shoulders & Triceps, Ab Ripper X
   _4 Yoga X
   _5 Legs & Back, Ab Ripper X
   _6 Kenpo X
   _7 Rest or X Stretch

By the end of this week, you should start to feel very strong and ready to pump more iron (or stretch more rubber)!

WEEK 8

RECOVERY AND AB FOCUS

DAY_1 Yoga X
   _2 Core Synergistics
   _3 Kenpo X
   _4 X Stretch
   _5 Cardio X
   _6 Yoga X
   _7 Rest or X Stretch

WEEKS 9–12

"No pain, no gain" is what this phase is all about. At this stage, you should be ready to leave everything you've got on your exercise mat. No holding back, no getting used to anything—this'll be the time to push to exhaustion and muscle failure on every single set! Let's drop the reps a little and try to fail at 10 to 12 reps on weighted movements. After 4 weeks of being completely hammered, your body wants to rest. So instead let's push your personal envelope and see what you've got. We want your best effort, each and every day! When the going gets tough, the tough get going; be at your best when your best is needed; take no prisoners . . . you get the idea. You've come this far—now let's put the X in "extreme"!

WEEKS 9 AND 11

DAY_1 Chest & Back, Ab Ripper X
   _2 Cardio X
   _3 Shoulders & Arms, Ab Ripper X
   _4 Yoga X
   _5 Core Synergistics
   _6 Kenpo X
   _7 Rest or X Stretch

WEEKS 10 AND 12

DAY_1 Chest, Shoulders & Triceps, Ab Ripper X
   _2 Cardio X
   _3 Back & Biceps, Ab Ripper X
   _4 Yoga X
   _5 Core Synergistics
   _6 Kenpo X
   _7 Rest or X Stretch

This week will give your body a chance to fully rest and transform before taking your "after" pictures.

WEEK 13

DAY_1 Yoga X
   _2 Core Synergistics
   _3 Kenpo X
   _4 X Stretch   *RECOVERY AND AB FOCUS*
   _5 Cardio X
   _6 Yoga X
   _7 Rest or X Stretch

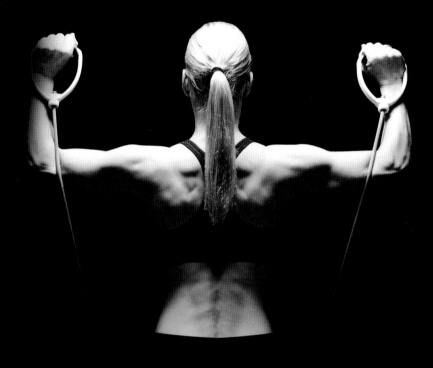

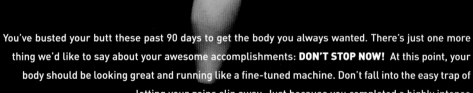

You've busted your butt these past 90 days to get the body you always wanted. There's just one more thing we'd like to say about your awesome accomplishments: **DON'T STOP NOW!** At this point, your body should be looking great and running like a fine-tuned machine. Don't fall into the easy trap of letting your gains slip away. Just because you completed a highly intense

FAST-FORWARD 90 DAYS

fitness program doesn't mean your work is over. We're not saying you need to perform a series of extreme workouts for the rest of your life, but you should continue with some type of fitness regimen that will maintain the results you've worked so hard to achieve.

The fact is, fitness is a lifetime challenge. By completing P90X, you just gave yourself one heck of a head start. In the following sections, we'll show you various ways to maintain and even build upon your P90X accomplishments.

ENOUGH LEARNING.

Just remember, when you're finished turning your body into a perfect physical specimen, there are a few important things you still need to do. The first of which is to take your . . .

"After" Photos: With your awesome, jaw-dropping new physique, you'll probably want to give it the maximum exposure it deserves. We suggest that you visit **P90XHome.com**, or if you're a member of the Team Beachbody community go to **TeamBeachbody.com/P90X**, to post your pictures. Any other type of self-promotion, such as a full-page photograph in your local newspaper, is up to you.

"After" Body Measurements: Once you're done with the camera, it's time to get the tape measure back out and take those "after" body measurements. Record all the dramatic results in the "After Day 90" blanks at the beginning of this section, or if you're a member of the Team Beachbody Community, go to TeamBeachbody.com.

Final Fit Test: To most accurately determine the progress made in your strength, power, coordination, flexibility, and cardio endurance, be sure to perform this test under the same conditions and timeline as the Fit Test you took prior to day 1. Record your "After Day 90" results in the blanks provided in this section.

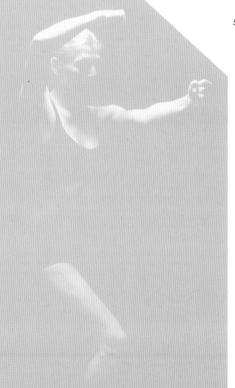

see you in 90 days.

Play the Million Dollar Body Game® for an opportunity to WIN BIG!

SUBMIT YOUR SUCCESS STORIES

P90X grads often say you can't put a price on the feeling of finishing the program, but now you *can* put a price on your transformation. Just submit your Success Story (including your "before" and "after" pictures, personal stats, and transformation story), and compete for prizes in Beachbody's Million Dollar Body Game.*

As you'll discover, P90X is not easy. So if you find yourself needing extra motivation to work out, eat right, and become a Success Story—now you have it. Get in the Game!

(Caution: We are not responsible for the new relatives you'll hear from when you win.)

*The Million Dollar Body® contest and sweepstakes are currently available only to U.S. residents. Certain limitations and restrictions apply. Please review the daily sweepstakes and monthly contest rules posted on TeamBeachbody.com for details.

To learn more about the Million Dollar Body Game, go to TeamBeachbody.com.

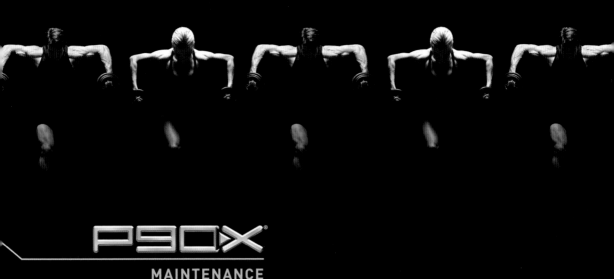

P90X

MAINTENANCE

P90X is an incredibly versatile program, and you can mix and match these workouts to fit just about any sports, recreation, or fitness routine you'd like to do next. Here are the basics, but for additional suggestions, check out the Beachbody Message Boards at **P90XHome.com**, or if you're a member of the Team Beachbody community, go to **TeamBeachbody.com/P90X**.

MIX AND MATCH

There's no problem continuing with P90X the same way you've been going at it. With the training block system, you aren't likely to plateau for some time yet. And with a little creativity, you never will!

If you want to challenge yourself further and go to the next level, incorporate the P90X Plus workouts.

_If you're happy with your results and would like to back off, try this:

Each week, do the Yoga X routine at least once. Also do Plyometrics, Core Synergistics, or Kenpo X once or twice a week.

To maintain your muscle mass, you can do just the first round of the resistance programs, since you get 80 percent of the benefit in a resistance workout during the first set. This rate isn't enough for you to make big gains, but it's enough to maintain your muscle mass for quite some time. This can cut the time of your resistance workouts to under 30 minutes until it's time to make another leap in your physical prowess.

LIFE AFTER P90X

P90X is a program that has prepared you for a life filled with possibilities. The completion of this program has provided you with the tools to take on almost anything. The intensity and variety of P90X has also given you the strength, balance, flexibility, coordination, and cardiovascular endurance to improve on any and all athletic activity. As a P90X graduate, you're motivated, confident, self-assured, and ready to attack any fear you might have had prior to starting this program.

The continuum of P90X is to explore the possibilities. The person you see standing in the mirror today is not the same person you saw on day 1. The person you are now is capable of so much more than the person who was just starting P90X. You decided, committed, and succeeded with P90X, so it's only natural to be curious about what else you can do and accomplish.

The truth about P90X is that there's no end. This program is an ongoing approach to staying in awesome shape. That doesn't mean you must continue to hammer out P90X workouts 6 days a week. It means that this is a fitness program that can be used for the rest of your life. It's a program that grows with you as you continue to explore and improve physically and mentally. If you're up for taking it to the next level, you can incorporate P90X+® workouts. Otherwise, P90X can be integrated into, combined with, and used to enhance everything else you're doing to stay in shape and enjoy your life.

Your choice to embark upon the P90X journey will have benefits that last a lifetime. Now it's time for your new journey to begin.

Congratulations on a job well done. Don't stop!

_TONY HORTON

The following section contains a complete and detailed listing of all the workouts in this program. You do not have to read this section to perform any of the P90X routines. You will, however, be asked to record important data (rep counts and weight amounts) on worksheets. You'll find that

WORKOUT GUIDE

recording this information is easy and extremely helpful toward charting your fitness progress. Free downloadable worksheets are available at **P90XWorkoutSheets.com**, or if you're a member of the Team Beachbody community, go to **TeamBeachbody.com/P90X**.

The detailed workout listings can also prove useful should you want to do the P90X exercises in your local gym, or if you need additional information about any of the workouts or individual exercises. And when you don't have access to a DVD player, you can perform the appropriate P90X workout straight from this book. Consider this section just another useful tool to help you maximize your results.

Everything depends totally on you and your individual goals. P90X is versatile. It will improve anyone's overall condition, but you can choose to tailor this program to gain mass, lean out, or maximize your strength. It's all a matter of setting

HOW MANY REPS SHOULD I DO?

your target number of reps, which will determine how much weight you use. Here's a quick rundown on what it means to "fail" at a given number of reps. (Simply stopping at your target number is not what we mean. Choosing a weight so you reach muscle failure at the right number of reps is what you're after.)

8–10 REPS =

*MUSCLE SIZE OR HYPERTROPHY_* In this range, you'll get maximum muscle growth. For those trying to achieve maximal size, this is your target area for every set in each workout.

12+ REPS =

*MUSCULAR ENDURANCE_* Some muscle growth will occur, but the volume of repetitions makes it self-limiting. You can build lean, strong muscles, but you'll never maximize your body's potential for size and strength in this realm.

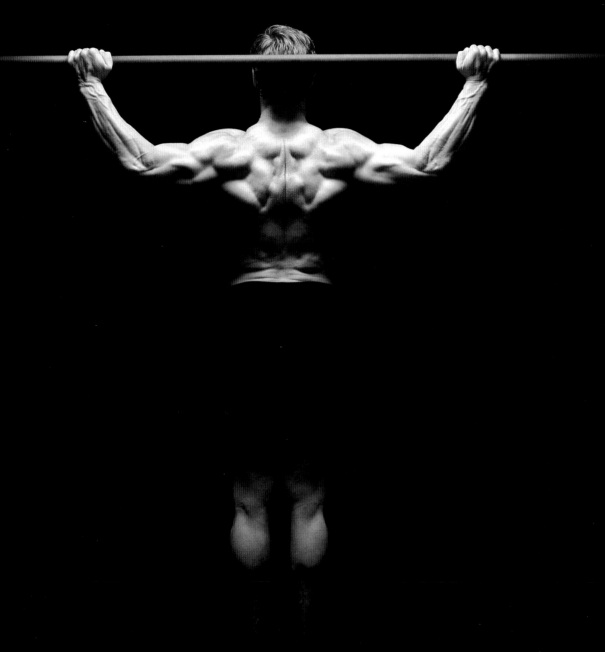

CHEST & BACK

Superset two of the body's largest muscle groups for a lactic acid bath like no other! You'll be fully pumped 5 minutes into the program, and your muscles will beg for mercy the rest of the way. Your body will learn how to keep it together under duress as you struggle to meet your target number of reps during round two. And if you feel a little queasy after your set, at least you'll know you're not alone.

LIGHT CARDIO WARM-UP AND STRETCH

[30 SECONDS] *March in Place*

[45 SECONDS] *Run in Place* – 15 seconds with knees up, 15 seconds with knees wide, 15 seconds with heels up.

[30 SECONDS] *Jumping Jacks*

[30 SECONDS] *Run Lunges with Alternate Arm Raises*

[6 REPS] *Side-to-Side Head Rolls* – Standing tall with arms at sides, reach to floor and roll head from right shoulder down to left shoulder and back.

[3 REPS] *Expand/Contract Chest-Back-Shoulder Stretch* – With feet wide apart, inhale while reaching arms up, reaching tall, then release arms downward, expanding the chest, reaching elbows behind you. Arms wide, fingers flexed.

[3 REPS] *Topas Shoulder Stretch* – In wide stance, start with hands in prayer position at chest. Inhale and open arms out straight to side, palms up, thumbs pointing behind you. Exhale back to prayer position.

Standing Side Stretch – Stand tall. Right arm reaches overhead while left arm is straight by your side. Tilt right pelvis out, reaching right arm toward opposite wall. Repeat other side.

[40 SECONDS] *Arm Circles* – Extend arms straight out at sides, palms up, fingers towards ceiling. Move arms in small circles 20 seconds clockwise and 20 seconds counterclockwise. Then position fingers down and rotate arms in larger circles for same amount of time.

Ballistic Stretches:

Huggers – Swing arms as if giving yourself a hug, alternating arm position every 20 seconds.
Swimmers – Simulate crawl stroke, then back stroke. Alternate arms.
Reachers – Standing with good posture, reach both arms up high and swing them back behind body as far as you can.
Shoulder/Triceps Combo Stretch – Extend left arm straight out. Grab upper left arm above elbow with right hand. Pull arm across body, bringing bicep in toward neck until you feel stretch in the shoulder. Hold for 20 seconds. Then raise bent arm overhead and, with opposite hand, grab elbow and pull arm back behind head. Repeat on other side.

Neck Stretch – Reach arm behind body (above waist) and grab wrist of that arm with other hand. Pull on arm while tilting head in opposite direction of arm you're pulling.

REP TIPS
During this workout, you'll perform a variety of push-up exercises. To get the most out of this routine, it's imperative to master the proper push-up form. You can avoid swayback, butt-rise, and improper head position by flexing glute (butt) muscles, gently tightening abs, and keeping the head and neck aligned with the spine.

1. When performing push-up and pull-up exercises, do as many repetitions as possible while maintaining good form throughout the movement. Try to set a rep goal prior to starting your set. For pull-ups, that goal should be somewhere between 8 and 15 reps.

2. The philosophy when performing exercises involving weights or bands is that 8 to 10 reps will build size, whereas 12 to 15 reps will create a slimmer, more toned look. There are only three exercises in this routine that call for the use of weights or bands.

3. Some people will find that at the beginning of this program, they may need to perform some or all of the push-ups on their knees for a greater range of motion. When you're capable of doing 12 to 15 reps from your knees with full range of motion, it's time to graduate to regular push-ups.

4. When performing pull-up exercises, a chair can be used either to help you perform a certain number of reps, or to take the place of a spotter when trying to knock out those last few reps.

Workout Tools: weights or bands • push-up stands • chin-up bar or band • chair • fitness guide and pen • water and towel

STANDARD PUSH-UP
1

_Keep back and abs tight and lower straight body until it's a few inches from floor.

WIDE FRONT PULL-UP
2

_Grasp chin-up bar using wide grip (a few inches wider than shoulder width). Pull body up until chin clears bar, and lower body back down. Be sure arms are fully extended at bottom position. If necessary, modify with one foot on chair.

BAND MOVE: *From seated, standing, or kneeling position, use a wide grip and pull handles toward chest.*

MILITARY PUSH-UP
3

_Place hands directly beneath shoulders. Keeping arms and elbows tight against sides, perform standard push-up movement.

REVERSE GRIP CHIN-UP
4

_Grasp bar with palms facing body. Pull up until chin clears bar. Lower arms to full extension and repeat. If necessary, modify with one foot on chair.

BAND MOVE: *From seated, standing, or kneeling position with a palms-up grip, pull handles toward chest.*

MINI-STRETCH

_Two-minute towel and water break with ballistic stretches. Keep moving throughout all breaks.

WIDE FLY PUSH-UP
5

_Extend hands three inches wider on each side than standard push-up position.

CLOSED GRIP OVERHAND PULL-UP
6

_Palms out, narrow grip. Perform standard pull-up motion. If necessary, modify with one foot on chair.

BAND MOVE: *From seated, standing, or kneeling position, hold handles close with a palms-down grip and pull toward chest, keeping arms and elbows close to body.*

DECLINE PUSH-UP
7

_Feet elevated on chair, step, or bench.

HEAVY PANTS
8

_With one foot forward and bent knees, bend at waist, keeping back flat. Lift weights from forward foot up to waist, keeping elbows close to sides.

BAND MOVE: *Shorten band by twisting in small loop. Then step on center with front foot. Perform same movement as above.*

Note: Powerstands can be used for all push-up exercises, except Diamond and Dive-Bomber push-ups. Keep in mind that this is a "repeat" workout where you'll perform two rounds of this 12-exercise routine.

MINI-STRETCH

_Two-minute towel and water break with ballistic stretches. Keep moving throughout all breaks.

_Stirrers – Bend over and hang one arm straight down. Swing in a circular motion as if stirring a giant pot for 10 seconds. Alternate arms.

DIAMOND PUSH-UP
9

_From push-up position, bring hands together so thumbs and index fingers touch. Align hands directly below heart. Elbows will flare out during push-up.

LAWNMOWER [8 TO MAX REPS]
10

_Side lunge, rest elbow on knee, pull weight from floor to waist. Repeat on other side.

BAND MOVE: *Stagger feet on band with wide-leg stance and pull front handle in same motion as above.*

DIVE-BOMBER PUSH-UP
11

_Move from a Downward Dog position (with wide hands and feet) to an Upward Dog position (the exercise simulates going back and forth underneath a fence). To modify, do NOT go back underneath fence. Just return to Downward Dog position and go under fence forward.

BACK FLY
12

_Seated at edge of chair, lower rib cage onto upper thigh, reaching behind heels. Keep wrists inward and elbows out and pull weight up toward ceiling. Pinch the shoulder blades together at top of movement.

BAND MOVE: *Shorten band by twisting in small loop. While seated, straddle band at center with both feet. Raise handles in a crisscross motion to perform same movement as above.*

REPEAT

_Repeat exercises 1 to 12 but switch order of every two exercises. Sequence is now 2, 1, 4, 3, 6, 5, 8, 7, 10, 9, 12, and 11.

COOL-DOWN AND STRETCH

Ballistic Stretches:

Shakers – Shake out body.

Huggers – Swing arms as if giving yourself a hug, alternating arm position every 20 seconds.

Swimmers – Simulate crawl stroke, then backstroke. Alternate arms.

Standing Side Stretch – Stand tall. Right arm reaches overhead while left arm is straight by your side. Tilt right pelvis out, reaching right arm toward opposite wall. Repeat other side.

Wide-Feet Forward Hamstring Stretch – With feet wider than shoulder width, reach arms skyward, bending forward at waist. Hang forward with legs straight. Fold arms and rest head on them or just hang arms straight down.

Cat Stretch – On hands and knees (hands directly beneath shoulders and knees directly under hips), round back while exhaling and drop chin to chest. Reverse move, inhaling while arching back and lifting head.

Child's Pose – Sit on your knees, chest resting on thighs. Extend arms out in front of you with head on floor. For added side stretch, while reaching overhead, slide both hands to left, placing right hand over left. Repeat on other side with left hand over right.

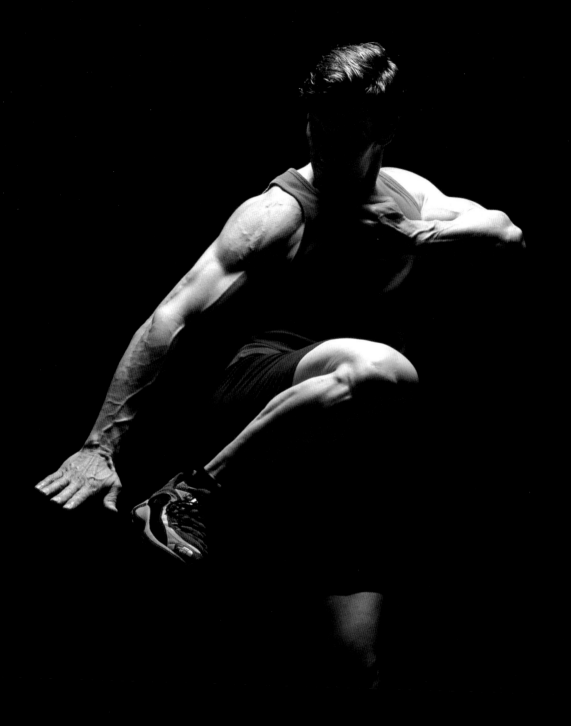

PLYOMETRICS

Plyometrics is a series of drills designed to connect strength with speed to produce power. Also known as "jump training," this technique emerged in Eastern Europe in the early 1970s. Coined by American track coach Fred Wilt, the term "plyometrics" derives from the Latin plyo+ metrics, or "measurable increases." Plyometrics training relates to any activity that requires speed and strength, as it improves your ability to run faster, jump higher, and maneuver in multidirectional sports. If your game involves a court, field, track, mat, pool, ring, rink, or mountain, plyometrics can help.

WARM-UP AND STRETCH

[60 SECONDS] *March in Place* – Rotate legs out for the final 30 seconds.

[60 SECONDS] *Run in Place* – Heels to buttocks for final 30 seconds.

[60 SECONDS] *Tires and Run Lunges* – Low-impact variety, rotating back and forth every 15 seconds.

[90 SECONDS] *Lunging Drills* – 2 forward, then turn and do 2 back.

[30 REPS] *Deep Prayer Squats*

Quad Stretch – While standing, grab left ankle with left hand and pull back toward buttocks, stretching the quad. Repeat on other side.

Hamstring Stretch – Standing with feet together, take large step forward, keeping heels aligned. Reach arms skyward and exhale forward over front leg. Repeat on other side.

> "The evolution of performance enhancement in today's world is truly amazing. There has been a virtual explosion in the number of trainers and coaches embracing plyometrics training as an integral part of their athletes' development."
>
> —Donald A. Chu, Ph.D., author of Jumping into Plyometrics

THE WORKOUT The key to avoiding injury during any plyometrics exercise is to ensure proper takeoff and landing. This technique can best be achieved by leaping off the toes and landing softly and quietly on the balls of the feet. Think Catwoman/Spiderman, not Frankenstein. Also be sure to wear good shock-absorbing sneakers and work out on a surface that provides plenty of cushioning. Trust us, the people in the apartment below will thank you, and so will your knees. If you adhere to this technique, you'll achieve the maximum benefits of this plyometrics workout, while at the same time minimizing your risk of injury. However, if you have chronic knee problems, we recommend that you substitute the less intensive Cardio X workout for this plyometrics workout. This is a "repeat workout," meaning you'll perform a sequence of four exercises, then repeat those same exercises before moving on to the next sequence.

Workout Tools: heart rate monitor • mat • stool or chair • water and towel

JUMP SQUAT
1 [30 SECONDS]

_With feet parallel and shoulder-distance apart, slowly (in a 4-count) ease into the bottom of a squat. At lowest point of the squat, quickly explode up, leaping off ground. Land gently and repeat.

TO INTENSIFY: *Maximize speed and reps and keep arms overhead.*

RUN-STANCE SQUAT
2 [30 SECONDS]

_Start with your feet in a stance that looks like you're about to run. The toe of the front foot should be aligned with the heel of the back foot. Perform 4 squats in this stance. After completion of the fourth squat, leap up, twist, and land facing in the opposite direction. Repeat.

TO INTENSIFY: *Increase speed and height of jump.*

AIRBORNE HEISMAN
3 [30 SECONDS]

_This is a lateral leaping exercise. Start with feet together and jump sideways. As soon as you land, bring opposite knee to your chest. Repeat back and forth.

TO INTENSIFY: *Grab bottom of foot with each hand. Strike the Heisman Pose.*

SWING KICK
4 [60 SECONDS]

_Stand directly behind a chair and lift one leg, then the other, back and forth over the chair. Modify by keeping knees bent over back of chair and control speed.

TO INTENSIFY: *Use a stool for more height and place hands behind head or straight up in the air.*

REPEAT PREVIOUS SEQUENCE
1 - 2 - 3 - 4

_30-second break. Use this time to grab some water, towel off if necessary, and keep moving to avoid cooling down.

SQUAT REACH JUMP
5 [30 SECONDS]

_This explosive move is performed by jumping straight up after a controlled squat.

TO INTENSIFY: *Deepen squat and fight for more height.*

RUN-STANCE SQUAT SWITCH PICK-UP
6 [30 SECONDS]

_Similar to a Run Squat, but jumping and changing direction after every squat. Try to touch the floor with every rep. Modify with minimal or no jump and no floor touch.

TO INTENSIFY: *Increase height and depth and touch the floor after every squat.*

DOUBLE AIRBORNE HEISMAN
7 [30 SECONDS]

_Just like the Airborne Heisman, but with 2 lateral tire steps instead of 1. Modify by stepping and not jumping sideways.

TO INTENSIFY: *Add more knee height in the middle of lateral leaps and strike the Heisman pose!*

CIRCLE RUN [30 SECONDS CLOCKWISE, 30 SECONDS COUNTERCLOCKWISE]
8

_While running around your rolled-up towel (or any other small item you won't twist your ankle on), try to keep your head and shoulders as steady as possible.

REPEAT PREVIOUS SEQUENCE
5 - 6 - 7 - 8

_30-second break. Use this time to grab some water, towel off if necessary, and keep moving to avoid cooling down.

JUMP KNEE TUCK
9 [30 SECONDS]

_Keep upper body relatively calm while jumping up and pulling your knees in toward your chest repeatedly. Use your hands as targets for your knees. Modify by lowering your hands, which decreases jump height.

TO INTENSIFY: *Raise hands to increase jump height and pick up speed.*

MARY KATHERINE LUNGE
10 [30 SECONDS]

_Starting in a forward lunge, jump straight up. Switch legs in mid-air, then land in a lunge.

TO INTENSIFY: *Extend arms straight up overhead.*

LEAPFROG SQUAT
11   [30 SECONDS]

_With legs wide, drop into a low squat. Keeping head and shoulders calm, jump/leap forward 2 times, then back 2 times. Modify by taking your time and not squatting too deeply.

TO INTENSIFY: *Deepen squat and increase speed.*

TWIST COMBO
12   [60 SECONDS]

_First 30 seconds: Jump up, keeping head and shoulders facing front while feet and knees twist right, then center, then left. Second 30 seconds: Spin body back and forth 180 degrees, changing directions after every rep. This exercise is about speed, not height.

REPEAT PREVIOUS SEQUENCE
9 - 10 - 11 - 12

_30-second break. Use this time to grab some water, towel off if necessary, and keep moving to avoid cooling down.

ROCK STAR HOP
13   [30 SECONDS: 15 SECONDS FACING LEFT, 15 SECONDS FACING RIGHT]

_Similar to Jump Knee Tuck, but instead of bringing knees to chest, you bring feet to butt. The Pete Townshend arm swing is a nice touch also. Not too high!

TO INTENSIFY: *Get up! Show 'em how to rock 'n' roll!*

GAP JUMP
14   [30 SECONDS]

_Leap/jump as far forward as you can, then turn around and do it again. It's very important to use your arms to swing you forward. Alternate lead leg when jumping.

SQUAT JACK
15   [30 SECONDS]

_Start with good old-fashioned jumping jacks in a squat position, then place hands behind head.

TO INTENSIFY: *Get down some more and extend arms straight up over your head.*

MILITARY MARCH
16   [60 SECONDS]

_Without bending your knees or elbows, march in place. Extend your arms as high and as far behind you as possible. Legs should be raised as high as possible in front of you. Right arm and left leg are up at the same time.

REPEAT PREVIOUS SEQUENCE
13 - 14 - 15 - 16

_30-second break. Use this time to grab some water, towel off if necessary, and keep moving to avoid cooling down.

RUN SQUAT 180 JUMP SWITCH
17   [30 SECONDS]

_In a Runner's Squat stance with lead hand touching the floor, jump straight up, turn 180 degrees in the air, and land facing in the opposite direction. Then jump back up and turn 180 degrees back to the original starting point. Turn left then back right for the first round, right and back left for the second. Modify by not touching the floor each time.

TO INTENSIFY: *Try to touch the floor every time.*

LATERAL LEAPFROG SQUAT
18 [30 SECONDS]

_The same as a Leapfrog Squat, but you move from side to side.

TO INTENSIFY: *Increase leaping speed, depth, and distance.*

MONSTER TRUCK TIRE
19 [30 SECONDS]

_Similar to Airborne Heismans, but traveling 4 big steps forward, then 4 back. No grabs or poses.

HOT FOOT [60 SECONDS: ALTERNATE
20 FEET AT 30 SECONDS]

_Alternate hopping from side to side, then from front to back, on one foot at a time. To modify, simulate slow jump-rope move.

REPEAT PREVIOUS SEQUENCE
17 - 18 - 19 - 20

_30-second break. Use this time to grab some water, towel off if necessary, and keep moving to avoid cooling down.

BONUS ROUND
21

Pitch and Catch [60 SECONDS]
Simulate a baseball pitching motion. Step on the rubber, raise knee, drive forward, and throw your best fastball. Be sure to follow through, squat down, and catch the ball. Do 30 seconds right-handed and 30 seconds left-handed.

22

Jump Shot [60 SECONDS]
First 30 seconds: Catch left and shoot right-handed. Second 30 seconds: Catch right and shoot left-handed.

23

Football Hero [60 SECONDS]
4 jukes forward (short and quick) and 6 high steps backward.

COOL-DOWN AND STRETCH

[30 SECONDS] *Easy Run in Place with Upper-Body Ballistic Huggers*

[30 SECONDS] *Easy Jump Rope* – Kick out one leg at a time.

[30 SECONDS] *Slow Marching with Low Kicks*

Wide Leg Bent-Over Hamstring Stretch – Standing with feet wide, bend forward at waist with straight legs. Place hands on floor or fold arms directly below head.

Downward Dog with Calf Stretch – In Downward Dog position, separate feet hip-distance apart. Slowly alternate bending one knee while straightening other leg, driving heel into ground.

Cat Stretch – On hands and knees (hands directly beneath shoulders and knees directly under hips), round back while exhaling and drop chin to chest. Reverse move, inhaling while arching back and lifting head.

Quad Stretch – While standing, grab left ankle with left hand and pull back toward buttocks, stretching the quad. Repeat on other side.

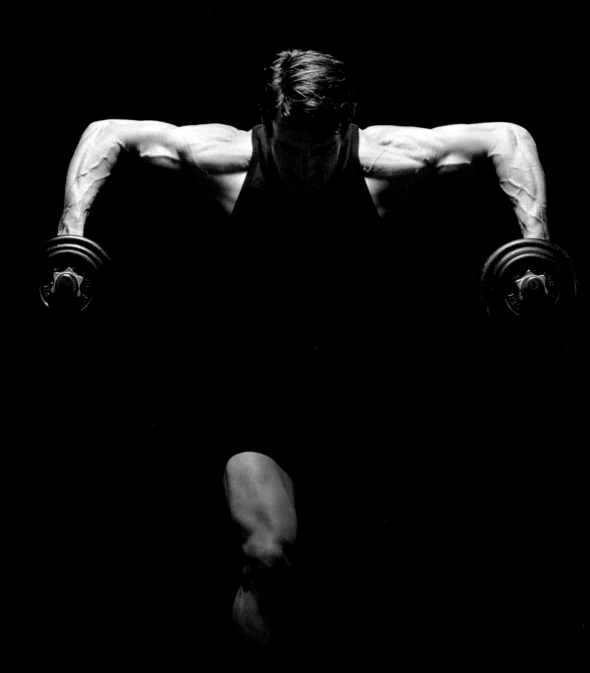

Applying the same principles as *Chest & Back*, you'll superset these muscle groups to exhaustion. As you'll be using smaller muscles, this might prove slightly less of a struggle—but that doesn't mean you won't be fully maxed when this workout is done. Just be sure

SHOULDERS & ARMS to keep your form during the latter part of the routine, when you'll be tempted to cheat your range of motion. Maintaining good form is critical for proper muscular development and preventing injury, so stay strict and get ripped!

LIGHT CARDIO WARM-UP AND STRETCH

[30 SECONDS] *March in Place*

[30 SECONDS] *Run in Place* – 15 seconds with knees up, 15 seconds with knees wide, 15 seconds with heels up.

[30 SECONDS] *Jumping Jacks*

[30 SECONDS] *Run Lunges with Alternate Arm Raises*

[6 REPS] *Side-to-Side Head Rolls* – Standing tall with arms at sides, reach to floor and roll head from right shoulder down to left shoulder and back.

[12 REPS] *Shoulder Rolls* – 6 back, 6 forward.

[2 REPS] *Crossed-Wrist Shoulder Stretch (front and back)* – Straighten arms down in front of body. Cross the wrists and clasp hands. Stretch back of shoulders (posterior delts) by bringing shoulders toward each other. To stretch front of shoulders (anterior delts), clasp hands behind back and squeeze shoulder blades together.

[3 REPS] *Expand/Contract Chest-Back-Shoulder Stretch* – With feet wide apart, inhale as you bring arms up, reaching tall, then release arms downward, expanding the chest, reaching elbows behind you. Arms wide, fingers flexed.

[40 SECONDS] *Arm Circles* – Extend arms straight out at sides, palms up, fingers toward ceiling. Move arms in small circles 20 seconds clockwise and 20 seconds counterclockwise. Then position fingers down and rotate arms in larger circles for same amount of time.

Ballistic Stretches:

Shakers – Shake out body.

Huggers – Swing arms as if giving yourself a hug, alternating arm position every 20 seconds.

Swimmers – Simulate crawl stroke, then backstroke. Alternate arms.

Reachers – Standing with good posture, reach both arms up high and swing them back behind body as far as you can.

Shoulder/Triceps Combo Stretch – Extend left arm straight out. Grab upper left arm above elbow with right hand. Pull arm across body, bringing bicep in towards neck until you feel stretch in the shoulder. Hold for 20 seconds. Then raise bent arm overhead and, with opposite hand, grab elbow and pull arm back behind head. Repeat on other side.

> *"There's something magical about well-built arms. They come in all shapes and sizes. However, when you see perfectly balanced biceps in front of rock-hard triceps, both supported by steel-ridged forearms, it's a vision you don't forget."*
>
> —Robert Kennedy, author of Awesome Arms

THE WORKOUT When performing exercises involving weights or bands, 8 to 10 reps will build size, whereas 12 to 15 reps will create a slimmer, more toned look. Use this philosophy when executing the following exercises.

Also keep in mind that this is a "repeat" workout, meaning that you'll perform a sequence of three exercises, then repeat those same exercises before moving on to the next sequence.

Workout Tools: weights or bands • wall • chair • fitness guide and pen • water and towel

ALTERNATING SHOULDER PRESS

1

_Standing military press using one arm at a time. Palms out at the bottom to palms facing inward at the top.

BAND MOVE: *Step on band with back foot. Perform same movement as above.*

IN AND OUT BICEP CURL

2

_Standard curl with palms-up grip. Bring weights back down and turn forearms out to sides for side curls. Bring weights back down. Rotate back and forth.

BAND MOVE: *Shorten band by twisting in small loop. Then step on center of loop with front foot and perform same movement as above.*

TWO-ARM TRICEPS KICKBACK

3

_Raise upper arms and keep at 90 degrees. Straighten arm to kick back the dumbbell. Make sure elbows remain stationary.

BAND MOVE: *Step on band with front foot. Perform same movement as above.*

REPEAT PREVIOUS SEQUENCE

1 - 2 - 3

_30-Second Ballistic Combo Stretches:

Shakers – Shake out body.

Huggers – Swing arms as if giving yourself a hug, alternating arm position every 20 seconds.

DEEP SWIMMER'S PRESS

4

_Press dumbbells overhead in modified corkscrew motion. Start with palms in. While raising dumbbells overhead, turn wrists so palms face out at top of move. Mimic move in reverse on way down.

BAND MOVE: *Step on band with back foot. Perform same movement as above.*

TO INTENSIFY: *Add full bicep curl at the bottom of the move.*

FULL SUPINATION CONCENTRATION CURL

5

_Start with palms facing in and arms slightly extended in front of body, creating slight tension in shoulders. Curl dumbbells and rotate wrists so palms face directly toward shoulders at top of movement. Squeeze at the top. Alternate arms.

BAND MOVE: *Step on band with back foot. Perform same movement as above.*

CHAIR DIP

6

_Heels on floor, legs straight, hands at sides of body and on front of chair, lower body off chair and lift back up.

TO INTENSIFY: *Put feet on chair, and/or alternate leg raise every 5 reps.*

REPEAT PREVIOUS SEQUENCE

4 - 5 - 6

_30-Second Ballistic Combo Stretches:

Shakers – Shake out body.

Huggers – Swing arms as if giving yourself a hug, alternating arm position every 20 seconds.

UPRIGHT ROW

7

_Pull up dumbbells from thighs to below chin. Elbows are higher than hands at end of movement. Maintain exaggerated posture throughout the exercise.

BAND MOVE: *Step on band with front foot and bring handles together on the way up.*

TO INTENSIFY: *Move with 2-count hold and added weight and/or reps, depending on fitness goals.*

STATIC ARM CURL
8

_Hold one arm static at 90 degrees, while other arm does 4 reps. Alternate arms and repeat sequence.

BAND MOVE: *Step on band with back foot. Perform same movement as above.*

TO INTENSIFY: *Add extra round (4 reps hammer curls) each side.*

FLIP-GRIP TWIST TRICEPS KICKBACK
9

_Stand leaning forward and perform standard triceps kickbacks, changing wrist position from palms-up to palms-down while hands are closest to shoulder. Alternate wrist position between each rep.

BAND MOVE: *Shorten band by twisting in small loop, then step on center with front foot. Perform same movement as above.*

REPEAT PREVIOUS SEQUENCE
7 - 8 - 9

_30-Second Ballistic Combo Stretches:

Shakers – Shake out body.

Huggers – Swing arms as if giving yourself a hug, alternating arm position every 20 seconds.

SEATED TWO-ANGLE SHOULDER FLY [16 REPS]
10

_Sit straight up and perform standard shoulder fly. Then lean forward so lower rib cage comes in contact with upper thigh, and perform fly movement from that position. Note: Be careful not to turn the bent-over shoulder fly into a back fly.

BAND MOVE: *While standing, step on center of looped band with front foot. Perform same movement as above.*

CROUCHING COHEN CURL
11

_With or without support of a wall, crouch to perform curl. Place elbows just below knees and be sure to straighten arms completely at bottom of movement. You may alternate the right and left arm.

BAND MOVE: *Shorten band by twisting in loop. Then straddle it evenly with both feet. Perform same movement as above.*

LYING-DOWN TRICEPS EXTENSION
12

_Lie on back on floor or bench. Bring dumbbells on either side of head, in line with forehead, keeping upper arms and elbows stationary while extending lower arms skyward. Raise and lower weights from the sides of your head straight up and back down.

BAND MOVE: *Standing with back foot on band, extend arms straight up overhead. Keep elbows locked and slowly bring handles back down toward shoulder blades.*

TO INTENSIFY: *More weight/more reps, depending on fitness goals.*

REPEAT PREVIOUS SEQUENCE
10 - 11 - 12

_30-Second Ballistic Combo Stretches:

Shakers – Shake out body.

Huggers – Swing arms as if giving yourself a hug, alternating arm position every 20 seconds.

BONUS ROUND
13

In and Out Straight-Arm Shoulder Fly
Extend arms straight forward for first fly, then out to sides for second fly movement.

BAND MOVE: *Step on band with back foot. Perform same movement as above.*

14

Congdon Curl
Curl weights up in standard palms-up position. Then turn wrists inward to bring weights down in hammer position.

BAND MOVE: *Step on band with back foot. Perform series of palms-up, palms-down curls.*

15

Side Tri-Rise
Lying on right side, place right hand on left shoulder and left hand between armpit and chest. Push up, raising upper body off the ground. Lower body almost to floor, then repeat.

REPEAT PREVIOUS SEQUENCE
13 - 14 - 15

Ballistic Stretches:

Shakers – Shake out body.

Huggers – Swing arms as if giving yourself a hug, alternating arm position every 20 seconds.

Reachers – Standing with good posture, reach both arms up high and swing them back behind body as far as you can.

Stirrers – Bend over and hang one arm straight down. Swing in a circular motion as if stirring a giant pot. Alternate arms.

[12 REPS] *Shoulder Rolls* – Six back, six forward.

Standing Side Stretch – Stand tall. Right arm reaches overhead while left arm is straight by your side. Tilt right pelvis out, reaching right arm toward opposite wall. Repeat other side.

[3 REPS] *Expand/Contract Chest-Back-Shoulder Stretch* – With feet wide apart, inhale as you bring arms up, reaching tall, then release arms downward, expanding the chest, reaching elbows behind you. Arms wide, fingers flexed.

[3 REPS] *Topas Stretch* – In wide stance, start with hands in prayer position at chest. Inhale and open arms out straight to side, palms up, thumbs pointing behind you. Exhale back to prayer position.

Shoulder/Triceps Combo Stretch – Extend left arm straight out. Grab upper left arm above elbow with right hand. Pull arm across body, bringing bicep in toward neck until you feel stretch in the shoulder. Hold for 20 seconds. Then raise bent arm overhead and, with opposite hand, grab elbow and pull arm back behind head. Repeat on other side.

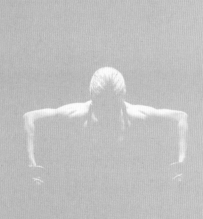

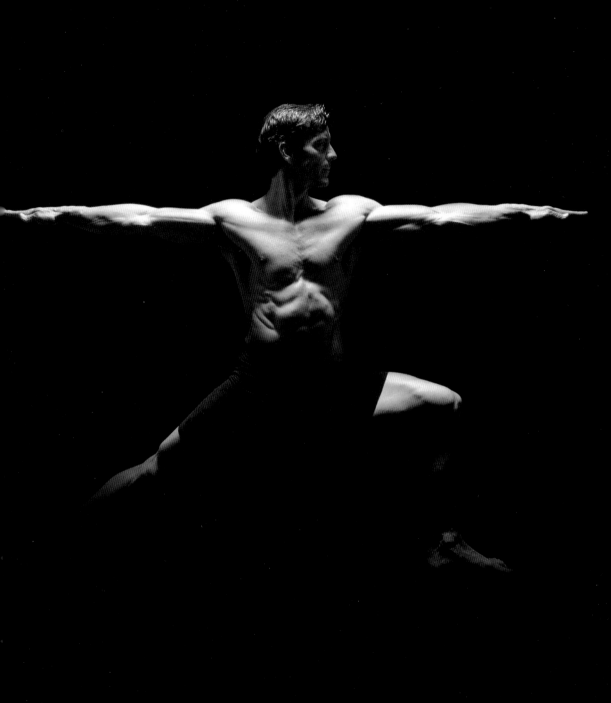

Namaste . . . welcome to Yoga X. The philosophy of hatha yoga, on which this program is based, is that the more you can focus on the breath through each pose, the less you'll notice the strain and discomfort. That's the goal of this workout. Although guys in particular may question

YOGA X   yoga's place in the X program, after one session they'll understand why this body-sculpting workout is a vital part of extreme fitness and an integral component of P90X. If you're new to yoga, this won't be easy—but you'll be amazed at your progress in just 90 days.

[5 BREATHS] *Mountain Pose* – Stand tall, feet together and parallel, arms straight by sides. Squeeze buttocks and tilt hips forward.

[5 BREATHS] *Wide Feet Forward Hamstring Stretch* – Standing with feet on either side of mat and folding forward at waist with straight or slightly bent legs, place hands on floor or fold arms directly below head.

TO INTENSIFY *Lock legs and flex quads.*

[5 BREATHS] *Wide Forward Bent-Over Torso Twist* – While in forward hamstring stretch, place left hand on floor (directly below your head), reaching right hand to the sky, with eyes on thumb. Repeat other side. Use yoga block if necessary.

TO INTENSIFY *Bend lower and reach higher.*

[5 BREATHS] *Split Leg Forward Hamstring Stretch* – Standing with feet together, take large step forward, keeping heels aligned. Turn left foot out with arms reaching skyward, exhale forward over straight front leg. Repeat on other side.

TO INTENSIFY *Lock legs and flex quads, reaching forehead toward ankle.*

[5 BREATHS] *Standing Side Stretch* – Stand tall with feet together. Right arm reaches overhead while left arm is straight by your side. Tilt right pelvis out, reaching right arm toward opposite wall, keeping eyes looking skyward. Repeat on other side.

[3 VINYASAS] *Astanga Sun Salutations* – Stand with feet together at front of mat, palms together at chest. Inhale, reaching arms up and into a slight back bend. Exhale, open arms, and swan dive forward, bending over legs. Place hands on floor next to feet. Inhale and raise torso up into flat back. Hold for beat, exhale forward, placing hands on either side of feet. Gently step or jump back into plank, then Chaturanga (bottom of push-up position). Inhale, pulling torso forward and up into Upward Dog pose. Then back to plank and perform a push-up. After push-up, exhale and raise hips and torso into Downward Dog pose. From Downward Dog, inhale, bending knees, looking between hands, and hop feet forward to hands. Keeping hands on floor, straighten legs. Keeping back and legs strong, inhale into reverse swan dive, ending with fingers skyward and with slight back bend. Repeat entire sequence two more times.

Downward Dog Calf Stretch – In Downward Dog position, separate feet hip-distance apart. Slowly alternate bending one knee while straightening opposite leg and driving its heel into the ground.

"If you look after the root of the tree, the fragrance and flowering will come by itself. If you look after the body, the fragrance of the mind and spirit will come of itself."

—B. K. S. Iyengar

THE WORKOUT

You'll want to perform your Yoga X workouts barefoot on a mat that provides plenty of traction. In other words, you shouldn't be slipping all over your mat. Also make sure you're in a comfortable, calm, and warm environment when performing this routine. If you can turn the phones off and avoid interruptions, you'll really get more out of this workout.

While you're in your yoga practice, focus on the following:

- Do not hold breath during postures. This can lead to strain. The eyes, ears, throat, and abdomen should remain relaxed.
- Avoid injury by not forcing the body beyond its capacity.

- Any real discomfort you feel in any posture should be temporary. Persistent pain is a sign of incorrect practice or some other physical problem.
- Create a calm and relaxing environment in which to perform the routine. (Turn off the cell phone for an hour.)
- Be patient throughout the early stages of your yoga practice. By the third month of Yoga X, you'll notice substantial improvements in your flexibility, balance, and coordination.
- As always, have water and a towel nearby, and respect the X. If you feel like you're out of control, take a break and regroup.

Workout Tools: mat • yoga blocks • water and towel

RUNNER'S POSE

1

_Bend over with legs split in a low forward lunge, front leg bent at 90 degrees. Knee should be over the ankle and back leg straight on the ball of foot. Fingertips barely touching the floor on either side of front foot. Lower torso toward floor and place both hands beside the instep of front foot or on the lower leg. Perform Vinyasa and repeat sequence on opposite side.

TO INTENSIFY: *Deepen lunge and lower torso until elbows rest on floor.*

CRESCENT POSE

2

_From Runner's Pose, raise torso straight up and reach hands skyward. Repeat on opposite side after Vinyasa.

WARRIOR ONE

3

_Same as Crescent Pose, except place back heel on floor. Perform Vinyasa.

TO INTENSIFY: *Deepen lunge and bring biceps close to ears during upward reach. Repeat on opposite side after Vinyasa.*

WARRIOR TWO

4

_From Warrior One position, extend front arm forward and rear arm backward. Arms should be parallel to the floor. Be sure hips and shoulders are in alignment. Repeat on opposite side after Vinyasa.

TO INTENSIFY: *Deepen lunge and work on opening hips.*

REVERSE WARRIOR

5

_From Warrior Two position, bend torso back toward rear leg, gently placing hand on straight back leg. Opposite arm, while turning palm up, reaches and extends overhead towards back wall. Repeat on opposite side after Vinyasa.

TO INTENSIFY: *Deepen lunge and extend reach without resting hand on back leg.*

TRIANGLE POSE

6

_From Reverse Warrior, straighten front leg, go to Warrior Two, and reach forward with front hand. Kick back hip out and lower front hand toward floor on inside or outside of front leg while raising opposite hand skyward. Look to skyward hand. Do a Vinyasa, then repeat sequence on opposite side.

TWISTING TRIANGLE

7

_From Warrior Two, straighten front leg, place hands on hips, and turn torso forward. Place left hand on back and reach right arm out, bringing hand to the floor while simultaneously raising left arm skyward. Use yoga block if necessary. Perform Vinyasa.

CHAIR TO TWISTING CHAIR (PRAYER TWIST)

8

_Feet together, bend knees 90 degrees, keeping back straight. Reach arms over head, sitting and pushing hips back toward heels. Come back up and stand tall on toes. Take a deep breath, then exhale and bring hands together while twisting torso to one side. At the end of twist movement, rest tricep of lower arm on opposite thigh while looking skyward. Repeat sequence on opposite side after Vinyasa. Perform Vinyasa (while in Downward Dog, raise leg, then swing knee forward up to forehead and hold; repeat three times).

RIGHT-ANGLE POSE TO EXTENDED RIGHT-ANGLE POSE AND GRAB

9

_From Warrior Two, same as Triangle Pose with front leg bent at 90 degrees. From Right-Angle Pose, extend skyward arm forward, creating a straight line from fingers to toes. Drop overhead arm behind back. Reach supporting arm under leg and clasp hands, turning torso away from floor and looking skyward. Repeat on opposite side after performing Vinyasa with three Knee Swing and Holds.

10 PRAYER TWIST FROM RUNNER'S POSE TO SIDE ARM BALANCE

_From Runner's Pose, twist torso toward lunging front leg, placing opposite arm on upper thigh. Place hands in prayer with elbow of other arm and eyes skyward. From Prayer Twist, lift and extend bent supporting leg straight out on top of other leg. Turn entire body sideways, raising arm toward ceiling while balancing on the other arm. Repeat sequence on opposite side after Vinyasa.

TO INTENSIFY: *During Prayer Twist, place hand on floor (instead of arm on thigh). Reach other arm skyward. Also, while in Side Arm Balance, raise upper leg.*

11 WARRIOR THREE TO STANDING SPLITS

_From Crescent Pose, lunge forward, shifting weight onto front leg and lifting back leg in line with torso. Straighten standing leg and reach arms straight ahead, parallel to torso and back leg. From Warrior Three, bend forward, raising back leg higher by opening hip. Bring hands to the floor, then grab standing leg with one or both hands while pulling head in toward leg.

12 HALF MOON TO TWISTING HALF MOON

_From Standing Splits (if standing on right leg), reach right hand forward near pinkie toe, simultaneously opening torso and lifting other arm skyward. Eyes are focused on skyward hand. Use yoga block if necessary. Switch hands and reach opposite arm skyward. Repeat on opposite side after Vinyasa. Perform your last Vinyasa for this workout.

BALANCE POSTURES

13 TREE [90 SECONDS]

_Stand on one leg, place foot on other leg on inside of thigh. Rotate knee of non-weight-bearing leg to side. Hold hands in Prayer position, then reach arms overhead. Repeat on opposite side.

14 ROYAL DANCER [90 SECONDS]

_Stand on right leg with left hand holding inside of left ankle. Push left foot out against hand, lifting leg. Tilt at waist while simultaneously raising right arm out in front of body. Keep palm skyward. Repeat on opposite side.

TO INTENSIFY: *Increase leg lift and lean forward.*

15 STANDING LEG EXTENSION [30 SECONDS]

_Balancing on one leg, raise opposite knee up as high as possible, then extend raised leg straight out and support by placing hand under thigh.

TO INTENSIFY: *Grasp big toe and extend leg to front. Keep both legs straight.*

FLOOR WORK

16 CRANE (PRE-HANDSTAND) [60 SECONDS]

_From a crouched position, place hands on floor, shoulder-distance apart, and open knees wider than elbows. Press inside of knees against upper arms and shift weight onto hands, lifting legs off ground. Focus on removing balancing foot from floor.

TO INTENSIFY: *Big toes gently touching each other.*

17 SEATED SPINAL STRETCH [5 BREATHS EACH SIDE]

_In seated position, pull right heel into left buttock and let knee drop to floor. Place left foot on floor on right side of right knee. Reach right hand skyward, place left hand on floor directly behind you. Twist torso to left and drop right elbow to the side of left thigh. On exhale, twist torso and head to left, while driving right elbow into thigh, keeping fingers skyward. Make sure head is up.

18 CAT STRETCH [9 REPS]

_On hands and knees with hands directly beneath shoulders and knees directly under hips, round back while exhaling and drop chin to chest. Reverse move, inhaling while arching back and lifting head.

FROG
19 [60 SECONDS]

_On hands and knees, spread legs wide, keeping lower legs in parallel position (90 degrees at hips and knees). Lower upper body down toward floor while gently pressing hips backward. Modify intensity by resting on forearms.

TO INTENSIFY: *Pelvis on floor. Forget it, guys.*

BRIDGE OR WHEEL
20 [5 BREATHS]

_While lying on your back, bend your knees, placing your feet on floor hip-distance apart with heels close to buttocks. Tilt pelvis skyward while clasping hands and straightening arms beneath you.

TO INTENSIFY: *From starting Bridge Pose, place hands on floor on each side of head (fingers towards shoulders) and begin to straighten arms and legs into back bend. To really intensify, while in Wheel, straighten arms and raise one leg to the sky.*

PLOUGH INTO SHOULDER STAND W/LEG VARIATIONS INTO PLOUGH
21

_Roll onto upper back, raising hips, supporting lower back with hands while resting on elbows (focus weight on elbows more so than shoulders and neck). Straightening legs skyward, keep shoulders, hips, and legs aligned. Perform 3 leg variations from this pose:

1) Split leg: extend legs out as far as possible for inner thigh stretch.

2) Inverted cobbler: soles of feet together, bend knees and open hips.

3) Scissor Splits: drop right leg over head with toes barely touching floor. Left leg remains straight up. Hold for 3 breaths. Repeat on other side.

After completing both sides of Scissor Splits, drop both feet to the floor. Final move of sequence is bending knees to ears. Come out of this pose by gently unrolling slowly from top of spine to lower spine.

TO INTENSIFY: *Focus on spine alignment during Shoulder Stand and increasing range of motion during leg variations.*

TABLE
22 [5 BREATHS]

_From a seated position, place palms on floor beneath shoulders, fingers facing forward. Bend knees with feet on floor, hip-width apart. Lift your body and drive pelvis skyward. Keep elbows locked, torso parallel to the floor and knees over ankles. Keep chin tucked into chest.

TO INTENSIFY: *Keeping spine aligned, tilt head back and look straight up.*

COBBLER POSE
23 [60 SECONDS]

_Seated with soles together and knees out to sides, grasp feet in close to hips. Pull feet in, stretching up with straight back (use towel under feet to alleviate ankle pain). Do 30 seconds with a flat back and 30 seconds reaching arms forward.

TO INTENSIFY: *Keep back straight while folding forward.*

ONE-LEGGED HAMSTRING STRETCH INTO TWO-LEGGED HAMSTRING STRETCH
24

_While seated, extend right leg out in front of you, bend left knee out to side placing left foot on inner thigh. Bend torso from hips over extended leg and clasp foot with both hands. Repeat other side.

Part 2: Straighten both legs for Two-Legged Forward Bend and repeat stretch. Grab as low as possible on leg or wrap towel around foot to assist stretch.

TO INTENSIFY: *Use yoga block for extended stretch.*

TOUCH THE SKY
25 [30 SECONDS]

_On back, raise arms and legs straight up toward ceiling. Keep chin tucked into chest to protect neck.

TO INTENSIFY: *Increase height of feet and hands.*

BOAT
26 [30 SECONDS]

_Sitting up and balancing on tailbone, raise legs together while simultaneously reaching arms forward and up. Note: Keep chest up, back straight, and palms facing upward. Modify by holding legs up with hands.

TO INTENSIFY: *Maximize chest and leg height.*

HALF BOAT
27 [30 SECONDS EACH SIDE]

_Same as Boat Pose, but with one leg bent (foot flat on floor). All 3 variations have both arms extended forward and up. Repeat on other side.

TO INTENSIFY: *Close gap between upper body and straight leg.*

SCISSOR
28 [30 SECONDS EACH SIDE]

_Lie on back with arms straight out to sides and palms down. Lift right leg 1 inch off floor and lift left leg directly over head, creating an "L" shape. Be sure to keep back flat on floor. After 30 seconds, switch leg position and repeat. Modify by adjusting lower leg to accommodate back strain.

TO INTENSIFY: *Focus on flexing feet and straightening both legs.*

TORSO TWIST HOLD
29 [30 SECONDS EACH SIDE]

_Lie on back with arms out at sides. Lift legs skyward, and tilt them to the right at a 45-degree angle. After 30-second hold, slowly swing legs over to the left side and repeat hold. Modify by lessening the leg-to-body angle.

TO INTENSIFY: *Close gap between torso and legs.*

DEEP TORSO TWIST HOLD
30 [30 SECONDS EACH SIDE]

_Extend legs further out to side, a few inches off ground. Repeat on other side.

TO INTENSIFY: *Close gap between torso and legs.*

TOUCH THE SKY
31 [60 SECONDS]

_Same as first position, but this time gradually increase leg and arm raise every 20 seconds.

TO INTENSIFY: *Maximize height of feet and hands.*

SIDE TWIST
32

_Lie on back, bend right knee, and pull heel into buttocks. Place left hand on outside of right knee and pull across body toward floor while looking right. Repeat on other side.

TO INTENSIFY: *Keep knee and opposite hand on floor.*

GLUTE STRETCH
33

_Lying on back and pulling knee inward, place right ankle on left thigh. Reach right arm between right and left thigh. Reach left arm on outside of left thigh. Clasp hands around left shin. Lie back and pull left knee in toward shoulder. Repeat on other side.

HAPPY BABY
34

_Lie on back, bend knees, grab outside of feet, and roll torso side to side. Be sure to keep lower legs equidistant.

CHILD'S POSE
35

_Sitting on knees, fold body over legs and relax head and arms on floor. Relax arms alongside body, palms up or out front with palms down.

TO INTENSIFY: *For added side stretch, while reaching overhead, slide both hands to left, placing right hand over left. Repeat on other side with left hand over right.*

SHAVASANA (CORPSE POSE)
36

_Lie on back and release muscles in legs, allowing feet to open outward. Rest arms alongside body, turning palms skyward. Place head in neutral position. Close eyes and relax completely.

FETAL POSE
37

_Lie on side with knees bent up toward chest.

MEDITATION POSE (LOTUS)
38

_Sitting with ankles crossed and back straight, rest hands on knees, palms up. Close eyes and breathe deeply.

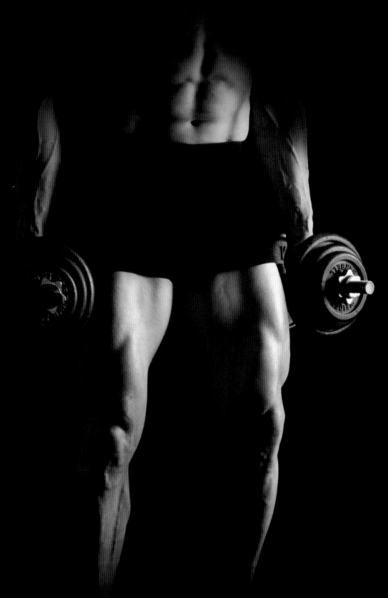

The Top-to-Bottom Resistance Calorie Burner. This workout went through more stages in its development than a prepubescent. Originally it was just a leg workout, but the pilot and test groups felt the program was too heavy on the legs and too light on, well, everything else. Tony can take

LEGS & BACK

a hint, and so was born this two-fisted, two-legged, total-body resistance blaster. While the main focus of the program lies in strengthening and developing the leg muscles (quads, glutes, hamstrings, and calves), there's also a handful of good old-fashioned pull-up exercises to give your legs a much-deserved break while you work the upper body.

LIGHT CARDIO WARM-UP AND STRETCH

[30 SECONDS] *March in Place*

[45 SECONDS] *Run in Place* – 15 seconds with knees up, 15 seconds with knees wide, 15 seconds with heels up.

[30 SECONDS] *Jumping Jacks*

[30 SECONDS] *Run Lunges* – Low impact; straight arm or pull variety.

[30 SECONDS] *Side-to-Side Head Rolls* – Standing tall with arms at sides, reach to floor and roll head from right shoulder down to left shoulder and back.

[12 REPS] *Shoulder Rolls* – 6 back, 6 forward.

[30 SECONDS] *Crossed-Wrist Shoulder Stretch (front and back)* – Straighten arms down in front of body. Cross the wrists and clasp hands. Stretch back of shoulders (posterior delts) by bringing shoulders toward each other. To stretch front of shoulders (anterior delts) clasp hands behind back and squeeze shoulder blades together.

[3 REPS] *Expand/Contract Chest-Back-Shoulder Stretch* – With feet wide apart, inhale as you bring arms up, reaching tall, then release arms downward, expanding the chest, reaching elbows behind you. Arms wide, fingers flexed.

Ballistic Stretches:

Huggers – Swing arms as if giving yourself a hug, alternating arm position. 20 seconds.

Stirrers – Bend over and hang one arm straight down. Swing in a circular motion as if stirring a giant pot. Alternate arms for 10 seconds.

Wide Feet Forward Hamstring Stretch – From a wide stance, fold forward at waist with straight or slightly bent legs. Place hands on floor or fold arms directly below head.

Runner's Stretch – Bend over with legs split in a low forward lunge, front leg bent at 90 degrees, knee over the ankle and back leg straight on the ball of foot. Place both hands near instep of bent front leg and lower torso to intensify stretch. Move hands to both sides of front foot. Straighten front leg while simultaneously lifting toes of front foot off the floor. Move back and forth between these two stretches (holding/breathing for a 6-count) 4 times on each side.

[40 SECONDS] *Standing Quad Stretch* – Stand tall with knees aligned. Reach left hand behind body to grasp left leg, pull heel up toward buttocks until stretch is felt. Hold for 20 seconds and repeat on other side.

"This routine is money, because let's face it, pull-ups are the coolest of all exercises, and nothing can accessorize a great leg pump better than wide-grip pull-ups till failure."

—Steve Edwards, Beachbody know-it-all and rock-climbing god

PULL-UP TIPS To achieve maximum intensity during pull-ups, focus on setting a goal for the amount of reps you'd like to perform (anywhere between 8 and 15 reps would be a good target). Because pull-ups can be difficult for women to perform, most will need to modify these exercises by using a chair for assistance. Men will also find using a chair helpful to max out on those last tough reps. Finally, when performing a pull-up, be sure to straighten arms completely at the bottom of every rep, but don't try to bounce off the bottom.

Workout Tools: weights or bands • wall • chin-up bar or band • chair • fitness guide and pen • water and towel

BALANCE LUNGE
1   [25 REPS EACH LEG]

_Extend one leg behind you, and rest top of foot on chair. Lunge on your standing leg, keeping knee over ankle.

TO INTENSIFY: *Add light weights and increase range of motion.*

CALF-RAISE SQUAT
2

_Squat progressing into calf raise.

TO INTENSIFY: *Add more weight.*

REVERSE GRIP CHIN-UP
3   [30 SECONDS]

_With palms facing body (shoulder-width apart), perform standard pull-up movement. If necessary, modify with one or two feet on chair.

BAND MOVE: *From kneeling, seated, or standing position with a palms-up grip, pull handles toward chest.*

SUPER SKATER
4   [25 REPS EACH SIDE]

_Place all weight on one leg and slide other leg behind body in skater motion, with toe touch for balance.

TO INTENSIFY: *Go lower and avoid touching toe on floor between reps.*

WALL SQUAT
5   [90 SECONDS]

_Two positions: thighs just above parallel and thighs just below parallel to the floor. Alternate every 15 seconds.

TO INTENSIFY: *Add an extra 15 to 30 seconds.*

WIDE FRONT PULL-UP
6

_Grasp bar with wide grip (a few inches wider than shoulder width). Pull body up until chin clears bar, then lower body back down. Be sure arms are fully extended at bottom position. If necessary, modify with one foot on chair.

BAND MOVE: *From kneeling, seated, or standing position, pull handles toward chest with a palms-down grip.*

STEP BACK LUNGE
7   [15 REPS EACH SIDE]

_Holding weights, stand with legs together. Hold hands at hips and step one foot back into a lunge, keeping knee over ankle of front leg.

BAND MOVE: *Step on band with front foot and perform same movement as above.*

TO INTENSIFY: *Raise arms above head or hold weights at sides.*

ALTERNATING SIDE LUNGE [24 REPS]
8

_Stand with feet together. Alternate lunges from right to left.

TO INTENSIFY: *Increase depth of lunges and hold dumbbells at sides during lunges.*

CLOSED GRIP OVERHAND PULL-UP
9

_With palms out and a narrow grip, perform standard pull-up motion. If necessary, modify with one or two feet on chair.

BAND MOVE: *From kneeling, seated, or standing position, hold handles close with a palms-down grip and pull toward chest, keeping arms close to body.*

SINGLE-LEG WALL SQUAT
10 [60 SECONDS]

_With your back flat against a wall and thighs parallel to the floor, squat with one leg, then straighten other leg out in front of you. Alternate legs every 10 seconds.

TO INTENSIFY: *Exceed 90 seconds and win Wall Squat gold.*

DEADLIFT SQUAT
11 [20 REPS EACH LEG]

_Standing on one leg with other leg bent behind you, squat down and reach for the floor.

TO INTENSIFY: *Touch fingers to the floor on every rep without touching other foot to the floor.*

SWITCH GRIP PULL-UP
12

_Alternate grip every 2 reps from shoulder-width pull-up to shoulder-width chin-up. If necessary, modify by placing foot on chair. Caution: If using chair for foot support, be sure to maintain good balance on chair before performing hand switch.

BAND MOVE: *From kneeling, seated, or standing position, pull band towards chest with palms-up grip for 2 reps, then switch to palms-down grip for 2 reps.*

BALLISTIC STRETCH
[60 SECONDS]

_Use this time to grab some water, towel off if necessary, and keep moving to avoid cooling down.

THREE-WAY LUNGE WITH
13 **TWO-KICK OPTION** [30 REPS]

_Lunge in three different directions: to the side, at a 45-degree angle, and to the front. After each lunge, raise/kick lunging (front) leg in either a straight or ball kick. Do in 3 sequences of 5 per leg.

TO INTENSIFY: *Increase depth of lunge and maximize height of kick.*

SNEAKY LUNGE
14 [20 REPS]

_Lunge across floor while on toes. While in lunge, bring lower rib cage to upper thighs so upper body is lined up with back leg. Extend arms upward, creating a straight line with body and straight leg, then reach back. Once exercise begins, heels never touch the floor. To modify, keep arms behind and in line with straight leg.

REVERSE GRIP CHIN-UP
15

_With palms facing toward body (shoulder-width apart), perform standard pull-up movement. If necessary, modify with one or both feet on chair.

BAND MOVE: *From kneeling, seated, or standing position with a palms-up grip, pull handles toward chest.*

CHAIR SALUTATIONS
16 [2 REPS]

_Stand tall with knees and feet together. With your weight on heels and arms at sides, inhale while raising arms straight up to ceiling. Exhale and begin to bend at the waist with straight legs and swan dive to the floor. When fingertips make contact with floor, bend knees into deep squat position, then raise arms up over head as high as possible. Hold for 30 seconds.

TO INTENSIFY: *Deeper depth, dapper Dan, and dipsy Dolly.*

TOE-ROLL ISO LUNGE
17 [20 REPS EACH SIDE]

_Exaggerate lunge position to prevent added pressure on the knee. Push off ball of foot, rolling onto toe of straight back leg. Knee stays above or behind ankle, never extending over.

TO INTENSIFY: *Increase depth of lunge and add weight.*

WIDE FRONT PULL-UP
18

_Grasp bar with wide grip (a few inches wider than shoulder width). Pull body up until chin clears bar, then lower body back down. Be sure arms are fully extended at bottom position. If necessary, modify with one foot on chair.

BAND MOVE: *From kneeling, seated, or standing position, pull handles toward chest with palms-down grip.*

GROUCHO WALK
19   [45 SECONDS]

_In a low squat position, walk forward 4 steps, then backward 4 steps.

TO INTENSIFY: *Get a little deeper with arms in the air (add cigar).*

CALF RAISES
20   [75 REPS]

_Do 15 slow reps and 10 fast reps in each of three directions: toes out/heels together, feet parallel, toes in/heels out.

TO INTENSIFY: *Add weights.*

CLOSED GRIP
21   OVERHAND PULL-UP

_With palms out and a narrow grip, perform standard pull-up motion. If necessary, modify with one or two feet on chair.

BAND MOVE: *From kneeling, seated, or standing position, pull band toward chest with palms-up grip for 2 reps, then switch to palms-down grip for 2 reps.*

80/20 SIEBERS SPEED-SQUAT
22   [30 REPS PER LEG]

_Squat at high speed. Be sure to keep 80% of body weight on heel of one foot and 20% on tiptoe of other foot.

TO INTENSIFY: *Go airborne!*

SWITCH GRIP PULL-UP
23

_Alternate grip every 2 reps from shoulder-width pull-up to shoulder-width chin-up. If necessary, modify by placing foot on chair. Caution: If using chair for foot support, be sure to maintain good balance on chair before performing hand switch.

BAND MOVE: *From kneeling, seated, or standing position, hold handles close with a palms-down grip and pull toward chest, keeping arms close to body.*

COOL-DOWN AND STRETCH

Ballistic Stretches:

Shakers – Shake out body.

Huggers – Swing arms as if giving yourself a hug, alternating arm position every 20 seconds.

Reachers – Standing with good posture, reach both arms up high and swing them back behind body as far as you can.

Stirrers – Bend over and hang one arm straight down. Swing in a circular motion as if stirring a giant pot. Alternate arms.

[3 REPS] *Expand/Contract Chest-Back-Shoulder Stretch* – With feet wide apart, inhale as you bring arms up, reaching tall, then release arms downward, expanding the chest, reaching elbows behind you. Arms wide, fingers flexed.

Wide-Feet Forward Hamstring Stretch – From a wide stance, fold forward at waist with straight or slightly bent legs. Place hands on floor or fold arms directly below head.

Downward Dog with Calf Stretch – In Downward Dog position, separate feet hip-distance apart. Slowly alternate bending one knee while straightening opposite leg and driving its heel into the ground.

Kenpo Quad Stretch – Start on hands and knees. Pull right knee up and between hands, turn outer ankle out towards floor, and sit on ankle. Push left knee back away from body, grab left ankle with left hand, and pull back towards buttocks. Repeat on other side.

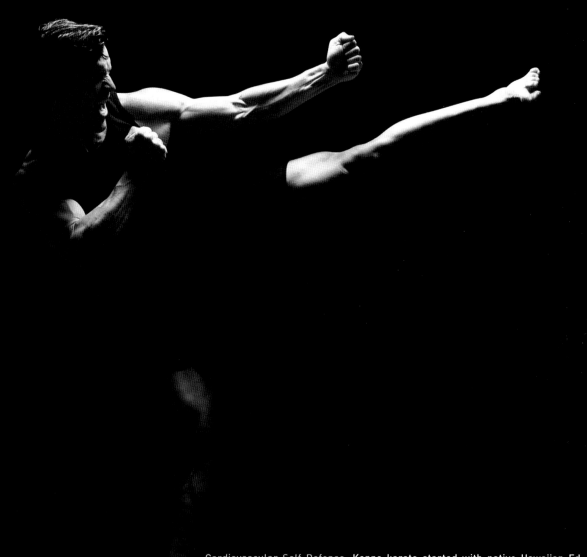

Cardiovascular Self Defense. Kenpo karate started with native Hawaiian Ed
Parker, Sr., who studied under martial arts masters William Chow and Lau
Bon. Parker's journey exposed him to the spectrum of martial arts forms
that originated in China, India, and Asia, which he combined to

KENPO X create Kenpo, a raw streetfighting style and the first American
system of martial arts. American Kenpo emphasizes the assets of gravity
and economy of motion—everything is used, nothing wasted. In the end,
one comes to know that the real weapon is not the fist or the foot, but the
whole body. Kenpo X was designed to give P90X users a high-intensity
cardiovascular workout loaded with fun, explosive combinations to improve
balance, flexibility, coordination, stamina, and confidence.

SAUNDERS STRETCH CYCLE

Most stretches are 20 to 30 seconds in length, or approximately 5 breaths each.

Straight-Arm Reaching Torso Twist – 1st motion: Wide feet, straight legs. Bend halfway down at waist and rotate torso from left to right side.

2nd motion: Bend all the way down to feet and rotate torso from left to right side.

3rd motion: Bend halfway down at waist and rotate torso from right to left side.

4th motion: Bend all the way down to feet and rotate torso from right to left side.

Prayer Squat – With heels under hips, rock back and forth in a Forward-Facing Side Lunge with palms on floor.

Forward-Facing Side Lunge – Sitting up in Prayer position, raise up on ball of foot.

Extreme Side Lunge – Place hands on floor on either side of straight leg. Take 3 breaths and turn into a Runner's Pose.

Kneeling Lunge/Reaching Arch Stretch – From Runner's Pose, place back knee on floor. Extend arms straight up and look up between hands. Then lift knee up from ground and go into Crescent Pose, to Prayer Twist, and finally back to Prayer Squat. Repeat sequence on opposite side, starting from Prayer Squat position.

Hip-Width Forward Hamstring Stretch – With feet parallel and shoulder-distance apart, bend forward at waist and fold arms. Then lower head and place forehead on forearms. Slowly roll out of stretch, then lie on back.

Lying Hamstring Stretch – Raise one leg straight up and grab hamstring (try to keep leg as straight as possible). Then grab calf, followed by toes (if you can). Then keep leg straight while extending out to side. Then bend and pull knee back in toward armpit and lower leg to start position. Repeat with opposite leg.

Pigeon into Kenpo Quad Stretch – Rest weight on outside of left leg and allow body to collapse forward. Reach behind and grab foot, and pull toward buttocks. Repeat on opposite side.

Frog – Still on hands and knees, spread legs wide, keeping lower legs in parallel position. Lower upper body down toward floor while gently pressing hips backward. Modify intensity by resting on forearms.

Cobra to Downward Dog with Calf Stretch – Start in Upward Dog position, but thighs should be resting on the floor. Float into Downward Dog and slowly alternate bending one knee while straightening opposite leg and driving its heel into the ground.

THE WORKOUT

Remember, every punch and every kick starts in a standard Fighter's Stance, except when directed to stand in Horse Stance. If you don't know what Horse Stance is, you need to watch this video! Additionally, whenever throwing any punches or kicks, be careful not to hyperextend (snap) your arms and legs. Be kind to your connective tissue—we're talking elbows and knees here. During any kicking sequence, be very conscious of hamstring flexibility or inflexibility. Don't try to kick out ceiling tiles because you think you're Jackie Chan or Bruce Lee, because your hamstrings will pay the price. During any block sequence, always remember that while one arm is blocking, the other fist recoils back to start position. Note: R = Right, L = Left.

Workout Tools: heart rate monitor • water and towel

TWIST AND PIVOT
1 [25 REPS EACH SIDE]

_While in a Fighter's Stance (knees bent, hands up), twist and turn torso so you're pivoting on both feet and driving hips with every big rotation. Repeat sequence on opposite side.

TWIST AND PIVOT WITH HOOK AND UPPERCUT
2 [25 REPS EACH SIDE]

_Same as Twist and Pivot, but adding Hooks and Uppercut punches. Repeat sequence on opposite side.

JABS
3 [20 REPS WITH 10 DOUBLES EACH SIDE]

_Start with right leg forward. Keep hands up and elbows down when throwing Jabs. Switch to left foot forward and repeat sequence on opposite side.

JAB/CROSS
4 [25 REPS EACH SIDE]

_Jab with forward arm, then throw a Cross Punch with back arm. Repeat sequence on opposite side.

JAB/CROSS/HOOK
5 [25 REPS EACH SIDE]

_Jab with forward arm, throw a Cross Punch with back arm, then Hook with forward arm. Repeat sequence on opposite side.

JAB/CROSS/HOOK/ UPPERCUT
6 [25 REPS EACH SIDE]

_Jab with forward arm, throw a Cross Punch with back arm, Hook with forward arm, then Uppercut with back arm. Repeat sequence on opposite side.

CARDIO BREAK

_Run in place for 30 seconds. Jump rope for 15 seconds. Jumping Jacks for 20 seconds.

STEP DRAG/HIGH-LOW PUNCH
7 [20 REPS WITH 10 DOUBLES]

_Step forward, drag, and throw high and low punch simultaneously. Repeat on other side.

JAB/CROSS SWITCH
8 [20 REPS]

_Switch feet quickly back and forth in Fighter's Stance between throwing Jab/Cross combinations.

HOOK/UPPERCUT SWITCH

9   [20 REPS]

_Same as Jab/Cross but with Hooks and Uppercuts.

KNEE KICK

10   [20 REPS WITH 10 DOUBLES EACH SIDE]

_While in Fighter's Stance, extend rear leg back, reach up with both hands (simulate grabbing someone's collar), and in one motion thrust back knee forward and up while simultaneously pulling hands to hips. Repeat sequence on opposite side.

BALL KICK

11   [30 REPS EACH SIDE]

_From Fighter's Stance, turn hips square and lift and kick back leg forward. Do 15 reps, then 15 more reps with greater height. Repeat sequence on opposite side.

CARDIO BREAK

_Run in place for 30 seconds. Jump rope for 15 seconds. Jumping Jacks for 20 seconds.

SIDE KICK

12   [30 REPS EACH SIDE]

_From Horse Stance, drag up left heel to right arch. Lean left, Side Kick right. Do 15 reps, then 15 more reps with greater height. Repeat sequence on opposite side.

BACK KICK

13   [25 REPS EACH SIDE]

_From Fighter's Stance with left foot forward, lean forward at waist, turn and look at target, and Mule Kick back behind you. Do 15 reps, then 10 more reps with greater height. Repeat sequence on opposite side.

THREE-DIRECTION KICK

14   [72 REPS]

_Kick 24 times each to the front, side, and back. The form that applies to these kicks separately still applies in combination. Always lean in opposite direction of every kick. This will allow you to achieve greater kick height and avoid injury.

TO INTENSIFY: *Avoid tapping the floor with foot between each kick.*

SIDE LUNGE WITH HIGH SWORD/LOW HAMMER

15   [15 REPS EACH SIDE]

_With hands up and feet together, lunge sideways, extending lead arm straight in karate-chop motion at neck level, followed by a Hammer Punch with the same hand. Repeat sequence on opposite side.

STEP DRAG/CLAW/LOW PUNCH

16   [15 REPS WITH 10 DOUBLES EACH SIDE]

_From Fighter's Stance, lunge forward, extending lead hand with open palm and clawed fingers at eye level. Then follow through with Hammer Punch, pulling clawed hand to hip. Repeat sequence on opposite side.

CARDIO BREAK

_Run in place for 30 seconds. Jump rope for 15 seconds. Jumping Jacks for 20 seconds.

HIGH BLOCK
17   [30 REPS]

_From Horse Stance with palms up and knuckles at hips, thrust or punch arm overhead as if to ward off downward blow. Alternate right and left arms. Each combo counts as 1 rep.

INWARD BLOCK
18   [30 REPS]

_From Horse Stance with palms up and knuckles at hips, thrust arm inward across face. Alternate right and left arms. Each combo counts as 1 rep.

OUTWARD BLOCK
19   [30 REPS]

_From Horse Stance with palms up and knuckles at hips, thrust or punch arm outward and away from body. Alternate right and left arms. Each combo counts as 1 rep.

DOWNWARD BLOCK
20   [30 REPS]

_From Horse Stance with palms up and knuckles at hips, thrust or punch arm downward and away from body. Alternate right and left arms. Each combo counts as 1 rep.

STAR BLOCK
21   [16 REPS]

_From Fighter's Stance using lead arm, the sequence is always block up, block in, block out, block down. Complete 16 cycles moving back and forth—4 forward and 4 back.

CARDIO BREAK

_Run in place for 30 seconds. Jump rope for 15 seconds. Jumping Jacks for 20 seconds.

FRONT SHUFFLE WITH
22   HIGH BLOCK/LOW PUNCH
[15 REPS WITH 10 DOUBLES EACH SIDE]

_Step forward and High Block simultaneously. Big hip turn and follow through with second Hammer Punch. Repeat sequence on opposite side.

KNEE/BACK KICK
23   [15 REPS EACH SIDE]

_While in Fighter's Stance, extend rear leg back, reach up with both hands (simulate grabbing someone's collar), and in one motion thrust back knee forward and up while simultaneously pulling hands to hips. Then lean and pivot on lead foot, followed by Side Mule Kick. Repeat sequence on opposite side.

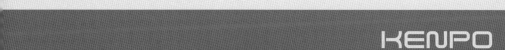

24 FRONT AND BACK KNUCKLES/ BALL KICK/BACK KICK
[10 REPS EACH SIDE]

_From Fighter's Stance, Back Knuckle front and back, followed by Ball Kick then Back Kick. Repeat sequence on opposite side.

25 HOOK/UPPERCUT/ LOW SIDE KICK
[10 REPS EACH SIDE]

_From Fighter's Stance with left foot forward, Hook left, Uppercut right, Side Kick right. Repeat sequence on opposite side.

26 ELBOW SERIES
[30 REPS]

_While in Horse Stance, drive elbow up, down, in, and out in a cross pattern (chin high). Alternate arms and don't start motion with second arm until first is completed.

27 VERTICAL PUNCHES
[100 REPS]

_In Horse Stance with palms up and fists at hips, alternate chest-high vertical punches. Increase speed every 10 reps.

CARDIO BREAK

_Run in place for 30 seconds. Jump rope for 15 seconds. Jumping Jacks for 20 seconds.

COOL-DOWN AND STRETCH

[30 SECONDS] *Easy Run in Place*

[30 SECONDS] *Easy Jump Rope with Ballistic Huggers*

[30 SECONDS] *Slow Marching with Low Kicks*

Wide-Feet Forward Hamstring Stretch – With feet wider than shoulder width, reach arms skyward, bending forward at waist. Hang forward with legs straight. Hands on floor or fold arms and rest head on them while rocking body from side to side.

Downward Dog with Calf Stretch – In Downward Dog position, separate feet hip-distance apart. Slowly alternate bending one knee while straightening opposite leg, driving its heel into the ground.

Quad Stretch – While standing, grab left ankle with left hand and pull back toward buttocks, stretching the quad. Repeat on other side.

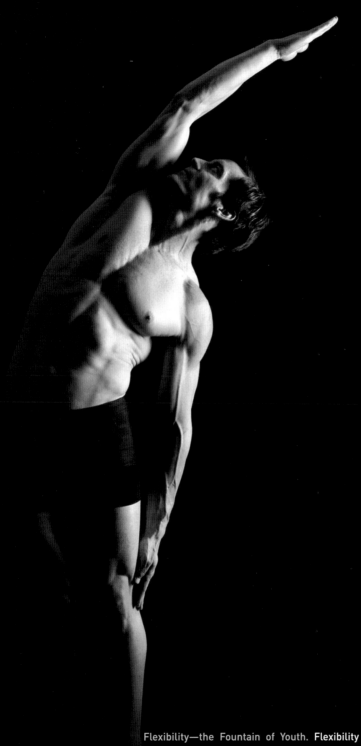

Flexibility—the Fountain of Youth. Flexibility training often takes a back seat to strength, speed, power, and cardiovascular endurance work, but the truth is that it can help you achieve a higher level of athleticism over a longer period of time. The reason so many fit people are inflexible is because they rarely ever

X STRETCH work at it! Ignoring this aspect of your training is a recipe for getting injured and hitting a plateau. It only stands to reason that the more you contract your muscles, the more you need to stretch them back out.

"Despite the recent bad press about stretching, we're keeping the faith. Yes, studies of high-level athletes have shown that stretching before maximal-effort events can reduce power production, limiting performance when it really counts. Our take: The next time you get invited to the Olympic trials, forget about stretching before the long jump. Before you work out at home, you want your muscles to be capable of a full range of motion."

—Michael Mejia, M.S., C.S.C.S

P90X is designed to use the whole body in very dynamic ways. This stretch sequence will help you prevent injury and avoid compromised results, which makes it an integral part of the program. This extensive full-body stretch uses disciplines from multiple sports: Kenpo, karate, and yoga.

Workout Tools: mat • yoga blocks • water and towel

SUN SALUTATIONS (VINYASAS)
1 [3 REPS]

_Stand at front of mat, with feet together and palms together at chest. Inhale, reaching arms up and into a slight back bend. Exhale, open arms, and swan dive forward, bending over legs. Place hands on floor next to feet. Inhale and raise torso up into flat back. Hold for a beat, then exhale forward, placing hands on either side of feet. Gently step or jump back into Chaturanga (bottom of push-up position). Inhale, pulling torso forward and up into Upward Dog pose. Exhale, pushing up hips and torso into Downward Dog pose. From Downward Dog, inhale, bending knees and looking between hands, and hop feet forward to hands. Keeping hands on floor, straighten legs. Keeping back and legs strong, inhale into reverse swan dive, ending with fingers skyward and slight back bend. Exhale to namaste. Repeat.

NECK STRETCH
2

_Reach arm behind body (above waist) and grab wrist of that arm with other hand. Pull on arm while tilting head in opposite direction of arm you're pulling. Repeat on other side.

BACK UP THE CAR
3

_Place arms straight out in front of you at shoulder height. Keep arms stable and turn head slowly to look over left shoulder. Repeat on other side.

HEAD ROLL
4 [6 REPS]

_Stand tall with arms at sides reaching to floor. Roll head from right shoulder down to left shoulder and back.

EXPAND/CONTRACT BACK-CHEST-SHOULDER STRETCH
5

_With feet wide apart, inhale arms up, reaching tall. Then release arms downward, expanding the chest and reaching elbows behind you. Arms should be wide, fingers flexed.

TOPAS SHOULDER STRETCH
6 [3 REPS]

_In Horse Stance, start with hands in Prayer position at chest. Inhale and open arms out straight to sides, palms up, thumbs pointing behind you. Exhale back to Prayer position.

WRIST-FOREARM FLEX STRETCH [20 SECONDS]
7

_While on hands and knees, point fingers out away from body. Lean slowly side to side 10 times, feeling the stretch. From same position, place palms flat on floor with fingers pointing backward toward knees. Slowly lean back until you feel stretch. Hold for 10 seconds.

DREYA FOREARM STRETCH
8 [2 REPS]

_Start with arms extended in front of you at shoulder height, palms up, fingers spread. Bend elbows, pulling hands in toward chest. Hold tension in hands and forearms as if pulling hands through wet cement. Finish by extending arms with fingers pointing downward and underside of forearms skyward.

ARM CIRCLES
9 [40 SECONDS]

_Extend arms straight out at sides, fingers toward ceiling. Move arms in small circles. Do 20 seconds clockwise and 20 seconds counterclockwise. Then position fingers down and repeat clockwise and counterclockwise movements for 20 seconds each.

SHOULDER-TRICEPS COMBO STRETCH
10

_Extend left arm straight out. Grab upper left arm above elbow with right hand. Pull arm across body until you feel stretch in the shoulder. Hold for 10 seconds. Then raise bent arm overhead and with opposite hand grab elbow and pull arm back behind head and hold for 10 seconds. Repeat on other side.

BALLISTIC STRETCHES
11

_**Huggers** – Swing arms as if giving yourself a hug, alternating arm position. Do for 20 seconds.

Reachers – Standing with good posture, reach both arms up high and swing them back behind body as far as you can.

Swimmers – One arm at a time, simulate crawl stroke 10 seconds, then backstroke 10 seconds. Alternate arms.

STANDING SIDE STRETCH
12

_Standing with feet together, place left arm alongside body and lift right arm overhead with palm facing floor. Open right side of rib cage. Repeat on other side.

ROLLER
13

_Lying on back, pull knees into chest by wrapping arms around legs. Tuck chin into chest and slowly roll back and forth, massaging the spine.

PLOUGH
14

_From Shoulder Stand, drop straight legs overhead until feet touch the floor. Then clasp hands and lay arms straight out on floor behind you. You may support yourself by placing hands on hips, using elbows for stabilization.

SEATED SPINAL STRETCH
15 [5 BREATHS]

_In seated position, pull right heel into left buttock and let knee drop to floor. Place left foot on floor, on right side of right knee. Reach right hand skyward and place left hand on floor directly behind you. Twist torso to left and drop right elbow to side of left thigh. On exhale, twist torso and head to left, while driving right elbow into thigh, keeping fingers skyward.

CAT STRETCH
16 [5 REPS]

_On hands and knees, place hands directly beneath shoulders and knees directly under hips. Round back while exhaling and drop chin to chest. Reverse move, inhaling while arching back and lifting head.

GLUTE STRETCH
17 [5 BREATHS]

_Lying on back and pulling knee inward, place right ankle on left thigh. Reach right arm between right and left thigh. Reach left arm on outside of left thigh. Clasp hands around left shin. Lie back and pull left knee in toward shoulder. Repeat on other side.

TO INTENSIFY: *Straighten leg.*

WIDE-FEET FORWARD HAMSTRING STRETCH
18

_With feet wider than shoulder width, reach arms skyward, bending forward at waist. Hang forward with legs straight. Fold arms and rest head on them or just hang arms straight down.

SIDE TWIST
19

_From Forward Fold, place right hand on floor below face and reach left arm up. Repeat on other side.

CAMEL
20

_While on knees, tilt pelvis forward and chest upward. Place hands on lower back while tucking chin to chest. One hand at a time, reach down and grab heel or bottom of foot. Then gently and slowly tilt head back. Note: Come out of this pose as slowly and gently as you went into it.

CAT STRETCH
21 [1 REP]

_On hands and knees, place hands directly beneath shoulders and knees directly under hips. Round back while exhaling and drop chin to chest. Reverse move, inhaling while arching back and lifting head.

BACK HERO
22

_Kneel with knees and feet slightly wider than hips. Slowly lie backward, sitting between feet. Support body on elbows or lie all the way back. Come out of this pose as slowly and gently as you went into it.

KENPO QUAD STRETCH
23

_Start on hands and knees. Pull right knee up and between hands. Turn outer ankle out toward floor and sit on ankle. Push left knee back away from body and grab left ankle with left hand, pulling back towards buttocks. Repeat on other side.

BOW
24 [30 SECONDS]

_Lying on stomach, bend knees, reach back behind body, and grab ankles. Arch back, lifting knees and chest off floor. Increase stretch and height by pushing feet against hands for added lift.

LOW SQUAT
25 [30 SECONDS + 10 BONUS SECONDS]

_Stand with feet shoulder-width apart or narrower, toes out. Squat down as low as possible, keeping chest and head up. Place hands in Prayer position. Use elbows to press against inner thighs to open hips. Gently rock back and forth.

FROG
26 [60 SECONDS]

_On hands and knees, spread legs wide, keeping lower legs in parallel position. Lower upper body down toward floor while gently pressing hips backward. Keep legs and hips at 45-degree angle. Modify intensity by resting on forearms.

SEATED SINGLE-LEG HAMSTRING STRETCH
27 [90 SECONDS]

_Extend right leg out in front of body with foot flexed. Bend left leg and turn knee outward, placing left foot on right inner thigh. Reach arm up overhead then bend at waist, collapsing torso over right leg. Repeat on other side. Always keep upper body relaxed, holding stretch for 45 seconds on each side. If needed, place yoga block at foot and reach around it for added stretch.

SEATED TWO-LEG HAMSTRING STRETCH
28 [45 SECONDS]

_From seated position, straighten both legs for two-legged forward bend and hold stretch. Grab as low as possible on the leg or wrap towel around foot to assist stretch. If needed, place yoga block at foot and reach around it for added stretch.

BALLISTIC HAMSTRING STRETCH
29 [10 REPS]

_Keeping both legs as straight as possible while flexing feet, scissor legs so that one leg is parallel with floor and other leg is pointing skyward. Switch leg position back and forth with 2-count between each switch.

SPLIT-LEG HAMSTRING STRETCH
30

_Standing with feet together, take large step forward with right leg, keeping heels aligned. Turn left foot out, with arms reaching skyward. Exhale forward over right leg. Repeat on other side.

TOE FLEXOR
31 [48 REPS]

_While standing, straighten right leg at comfortable height. Point and flex foot 8 times, then circle foot inward 8 times, then outward 8 times. Repeat on opposite side.

DOWNWARD DOG WITH CALF STRETCH
32 [20 REPS]

_In Downward Dog position, separate feet hip-distance apart. Slowly alternate bending one knee while straightening other leg and driving heel into the ground. Switch.

UPWARD DOG WITH ANKLE
33 STRETCH [60 SECONDS]

_From Upward Dog position, keep knees off floor. Rest body weight on top of feet, stretching ankles.

CHILD'S POSE WITH RIGHT
34 AND LEFT SIDE STRETCH

_Sitting on knees, fold body over legs and relax head and arms on floor. Stretch to right, then left by placing one hand over the other, then back to center. Relax arms alongside body, palms up.

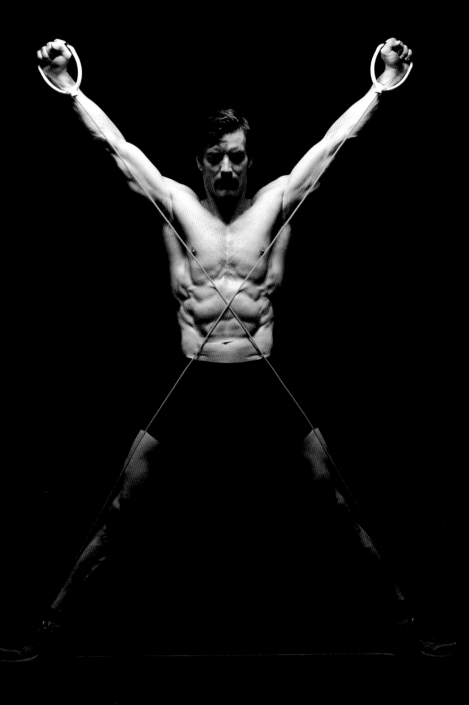

More Than Core. When it comes to maximizing your P90X results, the Core Synergistics workout is critical. That's because it focuses on strengthening the lumbar spine and trunk muscles, which are the foundation for all the other muscles in the body . . . especially during intense exercise. This **CORE SYNERGISTICS** routine recruits multiple muscle groups to build and support the core muscles, while at the same time conditioning your body from head to toe. Few people realize the vital role their core muscles play in everyday activities— which will give you even more of an edge.

LIGHT CARDIO WARM-UP AND STRETCH

[6 REPS] *Side-to-Side Head Rolls* – Standing tall with arms at sides, reach to floor and roll head from right shoulder down to left shoulder and back.

[3 REPS] *Expand/Contract Chest-Back-Shoulder Stretch* – With feet wide apart, inhale as you bring arms up, reaching tall, then release arms downward, expanding the chest, reaching elbows behind you. Arms wide, fingers flexed.

Ballistic Stretches:

Shakers – Shake out body.

Huggers – Swing arms as if giving yourself a hug, alternating arm position every 20 seconds.

Reachers – Standing with good posture, reach both arms up high and swing them back behind body as far as you can.

[60 SECONDS] *March in Place*

[45 SECONDS] *Run in Place* – 15 seconds with knees up, 15 seconds with knees wide, 15 seconds with heels up.

[30 SECONDS] *Jumping Jacks*

[45 SECONDS] *Run Lunges* – Low impact; straight-arm or pull variety.

[5 BREATHS] *Wide-Feet Forward Hamstring Stretch* – With feet wide apart, fold forward at waist with straight or slightly bent legs. Place hands on floor or fold arms directly below head.

[60 SECONDS] *Split-Leg Forward Hamstring Stretch* – Standing with feet together, take large step forward, keeping heels aligned. Turn front foot out with arms reaching skyward, exhale forward, and bend torso over front leg. Repeat on other side.

[40 SECONDS] *Standing Quad Stretch* – Stand tall with knees aligned. Reach left hand behind body to grasp left leg and pull heel up toward buttocks until you feel stretch. Hold for 20 seconds and repeat on other side.

REP TIPS

1. When performing push-up exercises, do as many repetitions as possible, maintaining good form throughout the movement.

2. The philosophy when performing exercises involving weights or bands is that 8 to 10 repetitions will build size, whereas 12 to 15 reps will create a slimmer/toned look.

Workout Tools: mat • weights or bands • plastic plate, cardboard square, or towel • water and towel

STACKED FOOT/STAGGERED HANDS PUSH-UP
1

_From standard push-up position, extend right arm out in front of body while positioning left hand tight beside rib cage (like a military push-up). Stack feet by placing right foot on top of left. Switch position of arms and legs after every fifth rep. Knee option if needed.

TO INTENSIFY: *Add raised-leg move.*

BANANA ROLL
2 [2 REPS]

_Start by lying on back with legs and arms extended straight out approximately 6 to 12 inches off the floor (biceps should be beside ears). Hold for 5 counts. Roll to side, keeping legs and arms extended and off floor. Roll to stomach, keeping legs and arms off floor. Hold for 5 counts. Continue to roll to other side, maintaining form, until ending up on your back in original start position. Repeat process, rolling back to start position.

TO INTENSIFY: *Increase maximum leg and arm reach.*

LEANING CRESCENT LUNGES
3 [24 REPS]

_Lunge forward at a 45-degree angle while extending arms straight out beside ears and then bringing them down again. Each arm position should form a straight line with your body. Alternate sides for each lunge.

TO INTENSIFY: *Increase depth of lunge and hold a 3- to 10-pound dumbbell in each hand.*

SQUAT RUN
4 [60 SECONDS]

_From a squat position, move arms back and forth as if running. Use light weights with modified intensity. Keep your core strong through entire sequence.

TO INTENSIFY: *Increase speed.*

SPHINX PUSH-UP
5

_Rest on forearms, elbows directly under shoulders. Hands should be flat on floor, shoulder-width apart. Body is supported by forearms and feet only. Press up off forearms until arms are straight. Go back down the way you came up. Focus on keeping entire body rigid throughout movement. Do as many as you can. To modify, perform on knees.

BOW TO BOAT
6 [5 REPS]

_Start on stomach. Reach behind and grab ankles to get in bow position. Lift chest and knees off the floor. Hold for 5 seconds, then roll onto back and extend arms and legs 6 to 12 inches off the ground. Hold for 5 seconds and repeat sequence.

LOW LATERAL SKATERS
7 [20 REPS]

_Start in side lunge position. Right knee is bent over right ankle while left leg is straight. While keeping fingertips on the floor, chest and head up and butt down, slowly shift body to opposite leg lunge position. Slowly shift back and forth 20 times. It's important to maintain wide width of lunge throughout movement.

TO INTENSIFY: *Lift straight leg a few inches off floor while in lunge.*

LUNGE AND REACH
8 [120 SECONDS]

_Reach down beside left foot and lift weight up with both hands. Extend arms fully over opposite shoulder. Bring back down to floor in same motion. After 30 seconds, repeat on opposite side.

BAND MOVE: *Place foot on band, reach down and grasp handle with both hands. Perform same move as above.*

BREAK AND STRETCH
[45 SECONDS]

_Use this time to grab some water, towel off if necessary, and keep moving to avoid cooling down.

PRISON CELL PUSH-UP
9 [8 REPS]

_From standing position, bend forward, placing hands on floor, then step or jump back into plank position. Perform a push-up, then bring right knee in toward chest, and put it back. Perform another push-up, and at top bring left knee in, then put it back. Do third push-up, then jump or step up to standing position. Entire sequence is 1 rep.

SIDE HIP RAISE
10 [30–40 REPS]

_Lying on side, rest bottom forearm on floor with elbow directly under shoulder. Place other hand on hip with elbow skyward. Lift body off floor with only forearm and outside of foot supporting body weight. Raise hips straight up in the air, pushing body past parallel. Keep hip off floor once you start exercise. Alternate sides.

TO INTENSIFY: *Raise nonsupporting leg throughout movement.*

SQUAT X-PRESS
11 [30 REPS]

_Holding light weights, start with feet wider than shoulder width and toes slightly pointed out. Go into a squat with chest and head up, and forearms on thighs. As you stand up, raise weights overhead into a wide shoulder press so your body forms an "X."

BAND MOVE: *Step on band with both feet wide. Grasp left handle with right hand and right handle with left hand. Extend arms up and out, pulling band across body and up toward shoulders, forming an "X" with the band.*

PLANK TO CHATURANGA RUN
12 [60 SECONDS]

_While in plank push-up position, bring knees in toward body as if running (more like slow jogging). Then lower body to Chaturanga position (just an inch off ground) and simulate a running (sneaking) crawl. Go from plank to Chaturanga every 10 seconds.

TO INTENSIFY: *Increase leg speed.*

WALKING PUSH-UP
13 [4 REPS EACH]

_Use towel for hardwood floor, sturdy cardboard for carpet, or just walk with your toes. Place feet on cardboard or towel and drag or walk legs across floor while walking with arms in plank position. Alternate forward and backward. Do this exercise slowly and methodically. Walk, don't run.

SUPERMAN BANANA
14 [60 SECONDS]

_Lying on stomach, extend legs and arms straight out in front. Try to get as much of your body off the ground as possible. Then roll to your back, keeping your legs and arms extended straight out, approximately 6 to 12 inches off the floor (biceps should be beside ears). Move back and forth between these two positions for 3 counts in each position. Always maintain a softball-size space between chin and chest.

TO INTENSIFY: *Increase height of arms and legs in both positions.*

LUNGE KICKBACK CURL PRESS
15 [20 REPS]

_Holding light dumbbells at sides (3 to 10 pounds), step forward into a lunge and lean torso forward so lower rib cage comes into contact with upper thigh. Raise elbows skyward as you bring weights toward shoulders. Keeping elbows stable, extend forearms straight back to raise dumbbells for a Triceps Kickback. Bring arms straight down to sides and lift rib cage off thighs. Maintaining your lunge, perform Bicep Curls, straight into Military Press, and then down into a Reverse Curl. When weights are down at sides, step out of lunge and repeat entire process on opposite lunge leg.

TOWEL HOPPERS
16 [60 SECONDS]

_Standing with both feet together, place a rolled towel on the floor parallel to your right foot. Keeping your knees together, hop over the towel (to the right) and land gently on your toes. Repeat in the opposite direction, hopping over the towel to the left. Always launch off your toes and land softly on your toes. To modify, step side to side over the towel.

TO INTENSIFY: *Bring knees higher and jump side to side across the towel faster.*

BALLISTIC STRETCH
17 [45 SECONDS]

_**Shakers** – Shake out body.

REACH HIGH AND UNDER
18   PUSH-UPS [MAX REPS]

_Combine a standard push-up with a one-arm balance. While in the one-arm balance, reach the top arm under body, near waist as far as possible, extending hip and buttocks into air, and then return arm back to top. Repeat on opposite side.

STEAM ENGINE
19   [50 REPS]

_Standing with feet shoulder-width apart, clasp hands behind head, keeping elbows wide. Alternate left elbow to right knee, while focusing on keeping head and chest up. Go from side to side. (It's like doing bicycle crunches while standing.)

DREYA ROLL
20

_From a standing position, squat down and place hands on floor. Roll from buttocks to back and kick legs straight up in air, keeping hands and forearms on mat alongside body. As feet come back to the floor, roll up and thrust arms forward to stand up. Try not to push off with your hands.

TO INTENSIFY: *Add jump at end of move.*

BONUS ROUND
20

Plank to Chaturanga Iso [60 SECONDS]
10-count in plank position, 10-count in Chaturanga position.

TO INTENSIFY: *Raise one leg on switch.*

21

Halfback [60 SECONDS]
Visualize running through wide tires, 4 tires forward. Then take 6 high steps back.

TO INTENSIFY: *Increase knee height and pace.*

22

Table Dip Leg Raise [60 SECONDS]
Sit on floor, feet parallel and shoulder-width apart. Place hands on floor with fingers toward your body. Raise one straight leg with toes pointing skyward. Lift buttocks off ground and drive hips up and away from floor as high as possible. Bending elbows, raise body up and down. Switch leg raise every fourth rep.

TO INTENSIFY: *Increase leg and hip height.*

DON'T JUST KIND OF DO IT.

[3 REPS] *Expand/Contract Chest-Back-Shoulder Stretch* – With feet wide apart, inhale as you bring arms up, reaching tall, then release arms downward, expanding the chest, reaching elbows behind you. Arms wide, fingers flexed.

Ballistic Stretches:

[15 SECONDS EACH] *Huggers* – Swing arms as if giving yourself a hug, alternating arm position every 20 seconds.

[15 SECONDS EACH] *Stirrers* – Bend over and hang one arm straight down. Swing in a circular motion as if stirring a giant pot. Alternate arms.

[5 BREATHS] *Wide-Feet Forward Hamstring Stretch* – From a wide stance, fold forward at waist with straight or slightly bent legs. Place hands on floor or fold arms directly below head.

[15 SECONDS EACH] *Downward Dog with Calf Stretch* – In Downward Dog position, separate feet hip-distance apart. Slowly alternate bending one knee while straightening opposite leg and driving its heel into the ground.

[2 REPS] *Cat Stretch* – On hands and knees (hands directly beneath shoulders and knees directly under hips), round back while exhaling and drop chin to chest. Reverse move, inhale while arching back and lifting head.

Kenpo Quad Stretch – Start on hands and knees. Pull right knee up and between hands, turn outer ankle out toward floor, and sit on ankle. Push left knee back away from body, grab left ankle with left hand, and pull back toward buttocks. Repeat on other side.

Glute Stretch – Lying on back and pulling knee inward, place right ankle on left thigh. Reach right arm between right and left thigh. Reach left arm on outside of left thigh. Clasp hands around shin of left leg. Lie back and pull left knee in toward shoulder. Repeat sequence on opposite side.

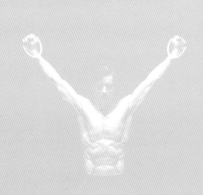

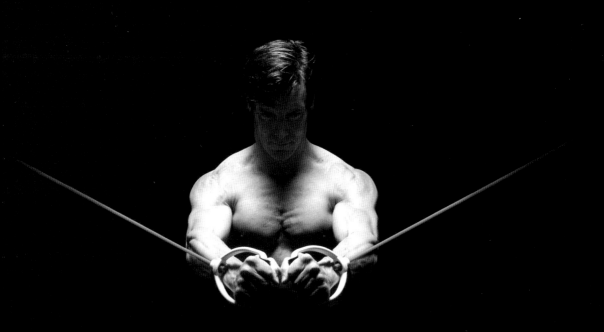

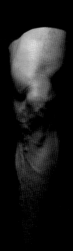

Do this upper-body blast a few times, and we guarantee that you'll never have to worry about anyone kicking sand in your face at the beach again. Even if you're not looking to bust out of your T-shirt, this series of exercises will leave you feeling super-chiseled on top. Just be prepared to "drop and give 20" on more than

CHEST, SHOULDERS & TRICEPS

one occasion. And ladies, if you keep your reps in the 12 to 15 range, you'll be sure to make the boys swoon. The good news: No curls or pull-ups today. The better news: There's every other move under the sun. So get ready to burn. Get ready to shred.

LIGHT CARDIO WARM-UP AND STRETCH

[30 SECONDS] *March in Place*

[45 SECONDS] *Run in Place* – 15 seconds with knees up, 15 seconds with knees wide, 15 seconds with heels up.

[30 SECONDS] *Jumping Jacks*

[30 SECONDS] *Run Lunges* – Alternate straight arms and pullers.

[6 REPS] *Side-to-Side Head Rolls* – Standing tall with arms at sides, reach to floor and roll head from right shoulder down to left shoulder and back.

[30 SECONDS] *Neck Stretch* – Reach arm behind body (above waist) and grab wrist of that arm with other hand. Pull on arm while tilting head in opposite direction of arm you're pulling.

[12 REPS] *Shoulder Rolls* – 6 back, 6 forward.

Shoulder Stretch (front and back) – Straighten arms down in front of body. Cross the wrists and clasp hands. Stretch back of shoulders (posterior delts) by bringing shoulders toward each other. To stretch front of shoulders (anterior delts), clasp hands behind back and pinch shoulder blades together.

[3 REPS] *Expand/Contract Chest-Back-Shoulder Stretch* – With feet wide apart, inhale as you bring arms up, reaching tall, then release arms downward, expanding the chest, reaching elbows behind you. Arms wide, fingers flexed.

[40 SECONDS] *Arm Circles* – Extend arms straight out at sides, palms up, fingers toward ceiling. Move arms in small circles 20 seconds clockwise and 20 seconds counterclockwise. Then position fingers down and rotate arms in larger circles for 20 seconds in each direction.

Ballistic Stretches:

Shakers – Shake out body.

Huggers – Swing arms as if giving yourself a hug, alternating arm position every 20 seconds.

Swimmers – Simulate crawl stroke 10 seconds, then backstroke 10 seconds (alternate arms).

Reachers – Standing with good posture, reach both arms up high, then swing them back behind body as far as you can.

ABOUT REPS   On push-ups and dips, there's no specified rep count. Just do as many as you can while maintaining proper form. When using weights or bands, follow the 8-to-10 rule if you want to build more muscle mass, and do 12 to 15 reps to develop longer, leaner, and slimmer muscles.

Workout Tools: weights or bands • push-up stands • plastic plate, cardboard square, or towel • chair • fitness guide and pen • water and towel

SLOW-MOTION 3-IN-1
1   PUSH-UP [12 REPS]

_Starting from a wide push-up position, lower body in 4 counts and raise in 4 counts. Repeat movements again in both military and standard push-up positions.

TO INTENSIFY: *Do some extra push-ups at the end (fast or slow).*

IN & OUT SHOULDER FLY
2   [16 REPS]

_Standing with straight arms, raise dumbbells straight out in front; bring down, then straight out to sides. Each movement equals 1 rep.

BAND MOVE: *Step on band with front foot. Perform same movement as above.*

CHAIR DIP
3   [30 SECONDS]

_Sit on edge of chair with hands holding front edge, legs extended straight out with heels on second chair. Lower body off edge of chair until upper arms are parallel to ground. Straighten arms and bring body back up to starting position.

TO INTENSIFY: *Alternate leg raise every 5 reps.*

PLANGE PUSH-UP
4

_Similar to Chaturanga/Military Push-Up, but the hands are placed farther back next to rib cage with fingers pointing out. At top of push-up, round your back as in Cat Stretch.

PIKE PRESS
5

_With feet on chair and hands on floor or push-up stands, lower upper body (at angle dictated by your level of strength) to simulate shoulder-press motion. Be sure to keep derriere in the air. Legs are straight so entire body creates a "V" shape. To modify, place toes on floor instead of chair. To further modify, perform without push-up stands.

SIDE TRI-RISE
6

_Lying on right side, place right hand on left shoulder near neck and left hand on floor close to chest, near armpit. Push up and straighten arm, raising upper body off the ground. Lower body almost to floor. Repeat on other side.

FLOOR FLY
7

_Military width to wide push-up width. At top of narrow push-up position, slide hand out while keeping the opposite hand stationary. When reaching wide position, perform push-up movement, then return to start (narrow) position and repeat. Do 4 reps right, 4 reps left. Note: Use a towel for hardwood floor; heavy-duty cardboard or plastic plate for carpet.

SCARECROW
8

_In staggered stance, hold light weights (5 to 10 pounds) in each hand, raising upper arms so they're parallel to floor with elbows bent at 90 degrees. Keeping elbows, wrists, and upper arms locked, rotate weights up and back as far as you can. Slowly return weights to starting position and repeat.

BAND MOVE: *Step on band with back foot. Perform same movement as above.*

OVERHEAD TRICEPS
9   EXTENSION

_Holding dumbbells, extend arms overhead. Keep upper arms stationary and elbows from flaring outward. Lower weights behind head, then straighten arms back up and repeat.

BAND MOVE: *Step on band with back foot. Perform same movement as above.*

TWO-TWITCH SPEED PUSH-UP
10

_Perform 4 fast and 3 slow standard push-ups. "Fast" are fast and furious, baby! "Slow" are 4 counts up, 4 counts down. Do as many as you can.

Y-PRESS
11

_Holding weights or band just above shoulders, press up and out slightly so at the top of the motion arms are in the shape of a "Y." Going too wide can result in injury, so don't do it.

BAND MOVE: *Step on band with back foot. Perform same movement as above.*

LYING TRICEPS EXTENSION
12

_Lying on back, bend one arm at elbow and bring weight close to floor on opposite side of your head, next to your ear (do not touch weight to floor). Straighten arm and drive fist toward ceiling, making sure to keep upper arm and elbow stationary throughout movement.

BAND MOVE: *While standing, straddle band with both feet. Perform same movement as above.*

BALLISTIC STRETCH

_Shakers – Shake out upper body. Use this time to grab some water, towel off if necessary, and keep moving to avoid cooling down.

SIDE-TO-SIDE PUSH-UP
13

_Starting from wide-feet, wide-hand push-up position, walk both hands to the right, perform push-up, then walk both hands to the left and repeat. Each sequence equals 1 rep. Modify by performing in standard push-up position. All three versions vary based on fitness level.

TO INTENSIFY: *Perform in Chaturanga (bottom of push-up position).*

POUR FLY
14

_Using light weight, raise arms straight out with dumbbells and tilt wrists to simulate pouring motion.

BAND MOVE: *Step on band with front foot. Do NOT use pouring motion. Instead, hold for a second at the top of movement.*

SIDE-LEANING TRICEPS EXTENSION
15

_Seated on chair, floor, or bench, lean left for right arm extension, pointing elbow straight up to ceiling. Lean on opposite side for opposite arm. Extend arm straight up, making sure to keep upper arm and elbow stationary throughout movement. Repeat on opposite side.

ONE-ARM PUSH-UP
16

_On knees (separated as far as possible), place push-up hand on floor below shoulder. Place other arm behind back. Go as low as you can and still get back up. Don't worry that you can't go all the way down. Partial range of motion still works with this exercise. Switch hands every other rep.

TO INTENSIFY: *Get off your knees. Show me what you got, Jack Palance.*

WEIGHTED CIRCLE
17 [40 REPS]

_Extend arms directly out to sides (shoulder height) and make slow circular motions with dumbbells. 10 forward + 10 reverse = 1 set. Repeat on opposite side.

BAND MOVE: *Step on band with extended front foot. Perform same movement as above.*

TO INTENSIFY: *Increase weight. Just a few more pounds will do it.*

THROW THE BOMB
18

_Raise arm overhead, and in a smooth controlled motion, extend upper arm forward as if throwing a football—but don't release! The range of motion is similar to Overhead Triceps Extension, but with a slight torso twist added. Repeat on opposite side.

BAND MOVE: *Step on band with back foot. Keep palm forward. Perform same movement as above.*

CLAP OR PLYO PUSH-UP
19

_Clap hands in midair between push-ups. Keep knees on floor if needed.

TO INTENSIFY: *Go airborne, baby.*

SLOW-MO THROW
20

_Holding weights at your sides, raise straight arms out in front of you at shoulder height. Keeping elbows from flaring, bend arms to bring weights beside your ears, keeping upper arms parallel to floor. Straighten arms out in front of you again, keeping arms parallel to the floor. Lower straight arms down to start position. Repeat for desired rep count. Be sure to maintain good form throughout. To modify, use hammer variation.

BAND MOVE: *Seated, lean back, keeping feet flat on floor. Step on band with both feet. Perform same movement as above.*

FRONT-TO-BACK TRICEPS EXTENSION
21

_While standing, hold weight in one hand with palm forward. Alternate moving weight in front of head, then behind head. Keep upper arm as stationary as possible throughout movement. Repeat on opposite side.

BAND MOVE: *Step on band with back foot. Perform same movement as above. Do 5 sets in front of head, then reposition band to perform 5 sets behind head.*

ONE-ARM BALANCE PUSH-UP
22

_Perform push-up, then twist up with one arm to perform one-arm balance. Look at the thumb of your skyward arm. Hold for a beat. Come back down and repeat on other side. Do one push-up between each balance.

TO INTENSIFY: *Raise same-side leg with arm.*

FLY-ROW-PRESS
23

_In a staggered stance, with knees slightly bent, perform fly (forearms should be parallel to the floor at top of movement). Complete first part of exercise, bringing hands back down to your sides, then perform upright row movement. Immediately drop elbows down, bringing weights to shoulders, and perform overhead press. Bring weights down to start position, using reverse curl for final move. Repeat sequence.

BAND MOVE: *Step on band with front foot. Perform same movement as above.*

DUMBBELL CROSS-BODY BLOWS
24

_Lie on back and hold light weight in each hand with arms bent and elbows close to sides. Alternate throwing pushes across the body without hyperextending your arms.

BAND MOVE: *While standing, step on band with front foot. Perform same movement as above.*

TO INTENSIFY: *Increase speed.*

TOO MANY PEOPLE STOP WAY BEFORE THEY SHOULD.

Ballistic Stretches:

Shakers – Shake out body.

Huggers – Swing arms as if giving yourself a hug, alternating arm position every 20 seconds.

Stirrers – Bend over and hang one arm straight down. Swing in a circular motion as if stirring a giant pot. Alternate arms.

Standing Side Stretch – Stand with feet together, place left arm alongside body, and lift right arm overhead with palm facing floor. Open right side of rib cage. Repeat on other side.

Wide-Feet Forward Hamstring Stretch – Standing with feet wide, fall forward at waist with slightly bent legs. Place hands on floor or fold arms above head.

Cat Back Stretch – On hands and knees with hands directly beneath shoulders and knees directly under hips, round back while exhaling and drop chin to chest. Reverse move, inhaling while arching back and lifting head.

Child's Pose – Sit on your knees, chest resting on thighs. Extend arms out in front of you with head on floor. For added side stretch, while reaching overhead slide both hands to left, placing right hand over left. Repeat on other side with left hand over right.

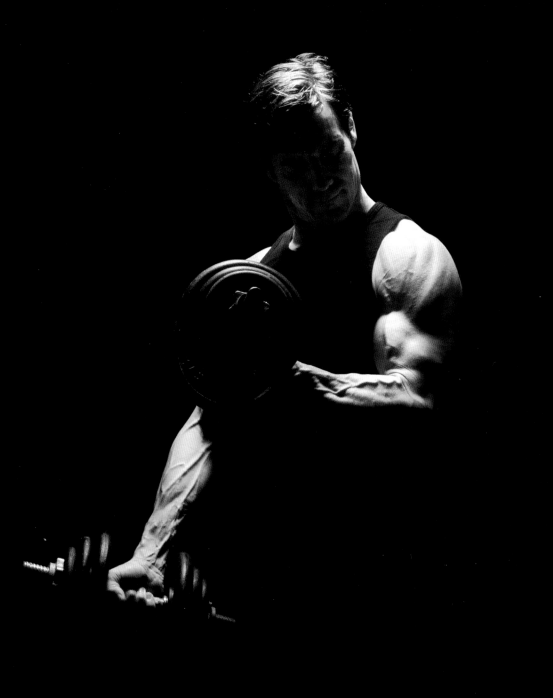

This program leads to some jaw-dropping biceps, also known as "guns" in the weight training world. While guys will definitely add major size to their favorite mirror muscle, this workout will also do wonders for women who just want to tighten and give definition to their back and upper arms. No matter what your

BACK & BICEPS   goals for this routine, you'll achieve them in dramatic fashion—just get ready to do a whole bunch of pulls and curls. When you're done, we guarantee you'll be your own "gun show."

LIGHT CARDIO WARM-UP AND STRETCH

[30 SECONDS] *March in Place*

[45 SECONDS] *Run in Place* – 15 seconds with knees up, 15 seconds with knees wide, 15 seconds with heels up.

[30 SECONDS] *Jumping Jacks*

[30 SECONDS] *Run Lunges* – Pulling motion and alternate arm raise.

[6 REPS] *Side-to-Side Head Rolls* – Standing tall with arms at sides, reach to floor and roll head from right shoulder down to left shoulder and back.

[12 REPS] *Shoulder Rolls* – 6 back, 6 forward.

Shoulder/Triceps Combo Stretch – Extend left arm straight out. Grab upper left arm above elbow with right hand. Pull arm across body, bringing bicep in toward neck until you feel stretch in the shoulder. Hold for 20 seconds. Then raise bent arm overhead, and with opposite hand grab elbow and pull arm back behind head. Repeat on other side.

[3 REPS] *Expand/Contract Chest-Back-Shoulder Stretch* – With feet wide apart, inhale as you bring arms up, reaching tall, then release arms downward, expanding the chest, reaching elbows behind you. Arms wide, fingers flexed.

[3 REPS] *Topas Stretch* – In Horse Stance, start with hands in Prayer position at chest. Inhale and open arms out straight to side, palms up, thumbs pointing behind you. Exhale back to prayer position.

[40 SECONDS] *Arm Circles* – Extend arms straight out at sides, palms up, fingers toward ceiling. Move arms in small circles 20 seconds clockwise and 20 seconds counterclockwise. Then position fingers down and rotate arms in larger circles for same amount of time.

Ballistic Stretches:

Shakers – Shake out body.

Huggers – Swing arms as if giving yourself a hug, alternating arm position every 20 seconds.

Reachers – Standing with good posture, reach both arms up high and swing them back behind body as far as you can.

Palm-to-Palm Shoulder Stretch (front and back) – Straighten arms down in front of body. Cross wrists and clasp hands. Stretch back of shoulders (posterior delts) by bringing shoulders toward each other. To stretch front of shoulders (anterior delts), clasp hands behind back and pinch shoulder blades together.

Important Note about Bands and Pull-Ups: When performing pull-up exercises using a band, be sure band is securely positioned in doorjamb.

THE WORKOUT Because this is a "no repeat" workout, each exercise should be performed so the last 3 reps are difficult. Use the weight you feel will best enable you to max out on the last 3 reps.

Keep in mind that 12 to 15 rep counts are for developing longer, leaner, and slimmer muscles, while lower (8 to 10) rep counts are more geared to build mass. The exception to the rule is with pull-ups. During these exercises, it's recommended that you just do as many pull-ups as you can during each set. Note: Because pull-ups can be a difficult exercise for women, most will need to modify these movements by using a chair for assistance. Men will also find using a chair helpful to max out on those last tough reps.

Workout Tools: weights or bands • wall • chin-up bar or band • chair • fitness guide and pen • water and towel

WIDE FRONT PULL-UP
1

_Grasp bar with wide grip (a few inches wider than shoulder width). Pull body up until chin clears bar, then lower body back down. Be sure arms are fully extended when in bottom position. If necessary, modify with one or both feet on chair.

BAND MOVE: *From seated position, use a wide grip and pull handles toward chest.*

LAWNMOWER
2

_In a side lunge position, rest left arm on left knee and pull weight with right hand from floor, straight up to waist. Perform desired rep count, then immediately repeat on other side.

BAND MOVE: *Step on band with front foot and perform movement above.*

TWENTY-ONE
3

_This is a three-part bicep exercise.

Part 1: Standing with weights at your sides, perform 7 half-curls (in final position, forearms will be parallel to floor).

Part 2: The final position of Part 1 now becomes start position. Perform 7 half-curls from this position to shoulders.

Part 3: Perform 7 full bicep curls.

BAND MOVE: *Straddle band with both feet and perform movements above.*

ONE-ARM CROSS-BODY CURL
4

_Alternating arms, curl weight across body and back toward shoulder of same arm. Repeat on opposite side.

TO INTENSIFY: *Add inward wrist twist.*

SWITCH GRIP PULL-UP
5

_Alternate grip every 2 reps from pull-up to chin-up. Switch with feet on ground. Caution: If using chair for foot support, be sure to step down during hand switch movement to prevent possibly crashing to the floor.

BAND MOVE: *From seated position, pull bands toward chest with palms-up grip for 2 reps, then switch to palms-down grip for 2 reps.*

ELBOWS-OUT LAWNMOWER
6

_Same move as regular Lawnmower, but with maximum elbow flare and palms facing back. Repeat on opposite side.

BAND MOVE: *Step on band with front foot and perform movement above.*

STANDING BICEP CURL
7

_Standing with knees slightly bent, curl both arms up at same time.

BAND MOVE: *Straddle band with both feet and perform movement above.*

ONE-ARM CONCENTRATION CURL
8

_In Lawnmower Stance with left knee bent and right leg straight, place left forearm on thigh above left knee. Grab dumbbell with right hand, placing upper arm at wrist of left arm. Left arm stabilizes right. Complete reps and repeat on opposite side.

BAND MOVE: *Step on band with front foot and perform movement above.*

CORNCOB PULL-UP
9

_At top of wide-grip pull-up, slide head to knuckles of right hand, then slide all the way over to knuckles of left hand. Come back to center. Move head away from bar, then back to center, then lower body to start position.

BAND MOVE: *From seated position, pull bands toward chest with palms-down grip. At end of movement, shift arms all the way out to the left side and then to the right. Bring back to center and repeat.*

REVERSE-GRIP BENT-OVER ROW
10

_With one foot forward and knees bent, bend at waist, keeping your back flat and palms facing forward. Reach straight arms toward front right toe, then pull weight up toward hips, driving elbows skyward.

BAND MOVE: *Shorten band by twisting in small loop. Then step on center with front foot. Perform same movement as above.*

OPEN-ARM CURL
11

_Turn forearms out to sides (palms up) and perform curl. Extend your arms as straight as possible at bottom of movement.

BAND MOVE: *Straddle band with both feet and perform movement above. To increase tension, spread feet wider apart on band.*

STATIC-ARM CURL
12   [16 REPS]

_Hold one arm static at 90 degrees while your other arm does 4 reps. Switch arms and repeat. Go back to the original side and repeat. Then switch again to perform the last 4.

BAND MOVE: *Straddle band with both feet and perform movement above. To increase tension, spread feet wider apart on band.*

TO INTENSIFY: *Add an extra round.*

BALLISTIC STRETCH
[90 SECONDS]

_**Huggers** – Swing arms as if giving yourself a hug, alternating arm position every 20 seconds.

Shakers – Shake out upper body.

TOWEL PULL-UP
13

_Put one hand on bar while other hand grasps a towel. Switch towel hand every 3 pull-ups. Come to floor to make proper adjustment. Note: A wet towel will provide a better grip.

BAND MOVE: *Put small towel through band handle. From seated position, pull toward chest. Switch towel to opposite handle every 10 reps.*

TO INTENSIFY: *Make towel adjustment without placing feet on floor. Good luck, towel boy (or girl).*

CONGDON LOCOMOTIVE
14   [40 REPS]

_With one foot forward and knees bent, bend at waist, keeping your back flat. Alternating arms, lift light to moderate weight from forward foot up to waist.

BAND MOVE: *Shorten band by twisting in loop. Then step on with front foot. Perform same movement as above.*

CROUCHING COHEN CURL
15

_Squat against wall with elbows just below knees. Extend arm fully at bottom of movement and squeeze at the top. If no wall is available, use regular squat position. Make sure feet are shoulder-distance apart.

BAND MOVE: *Shorten band by twisting in loop. Then step on it with front foot. Perform same movement as above.*

ONE-ARM CORKSCREW CURL
16

_Start with arms down at sides, palms back. Curl up one arm at a time and twist wrist inward.

BAND MOVE: *Straddle band with both feet and perform movement above.*

CHIN-UP
17

_Grasp bar with palms facing body. Pull up until chin clears bar. Lower arms to full extension and repeat.

BAND MOVE: *From seated position with a palms-up grip, pull handles towards chest.*

SEATED BENT-OVER BACK FLY
18

_Sit on the edge of a chair with your lower rib cage resting on your upper thighs. With feet together in front of body, reach behind heels, holding weights. Keep wrists inward and raise elbows up toward ceiling. Pinch the shoulder blades together at top of movement. Note: This exercise should be felt in middle of upper back, not in shoulders.

BAND MOVE: *Shorten band by twisting in loop, and step on it with front foot. Perform same movement as above.*

CURL UP/HAMMER DOWN
19

_Perform standard curl. At top, turn weight vertically and perform downward hammer curl. Repeat movement.

BAND MOVE: *Shorten band by twisting in loop. Straddle band with both feet and perform movement above. On the way down, use a palms-down grip to perform reverse curls instead of hammer curls. Do 2 regular curls, then 2 reverse curls.*

HAMMER CURL
20

_Same as standard curls but with palms facing inward.

BAND MOVE: *Shorten band by twisting in small loop. Straddle band with both feet, and with a palms-down grip, perform reverse curls.*

MAX REP PULL-UP
21

_Here's where you do your least favorite pull-up. Use a chair to get a few extra reps.

SUPERMAN
22

_Lying on stomach, extend legs and arms straight out in front. Try to get as much of body off the ground as possible. Heels and thumbs are skyward, arms and legs as straight as possible. Tilt head down slightly, keeping spine straight.

IN-OUT HAMMER CURLS
23

_Perform standard hammer curl. Bring weights back down and turn forearms out to sides for side hammer curl. Rotate back and forth.

BAND MOVE: *Straddle band with both feet and perform movement above. Use a palms-down grip to perform reverse curls instead of hammer curls.*

STRIP-SET CURL
24

_Perform 8 standard bicep curls with heaviest possible weight. After a 10-second break, lower weight by 5 pounds and repeat. Continue for a total of 4 rounds.

BAND MOVE: *Straddle band with both feet and perform movement above.*

YOU ARE WORKING SO BEAUTIFULLY HARD.

Ballistic Stretches:

Shakers – Shake out body.

Stirrers – Bend over and hang one arm straight down. Swing in a circular motion as if stirring a giant pot. Alternate arms.

[3 REPS] *Expand/Contract Chest-Back-Shoulder Stretch* – With feet wide apart, inhale as you bring arms up, reaching tall, then release arms downward, expanding the chest, reaching elbows behind you. Arms wide, fingers flexed.

Standing Side Stretch – Stand tall with feet together. Right arm reaches overhead while left arm is straight by your side. Tilt right pelvis out, reaching right arm toward opposite wall. Repeat on other side.

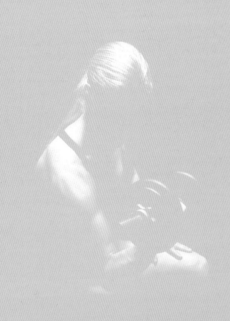

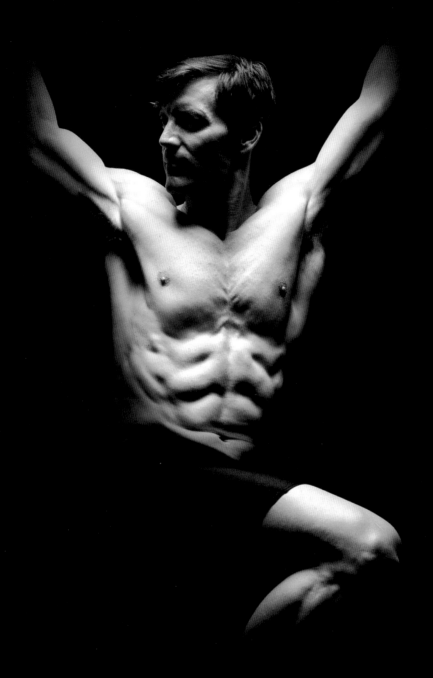

This is not your mother's aerobics class. Aerobic means "with oxygen." Cardiovascular endurance relates to your body's ability to efficiently transport oxygenated, nutrient-rich blood to working muscles. When training for strength gains, it's important to keep cardiovascular work under control or you could actually experience strength loss! In this workout, you'll keep your heart rate well below its anaerobic threshold—the point where strength gains are made and muscle fiber is broken down. Instead, you'll sweat comfortably as your body pumps oxygenated blood through your system, flushing out lactic acid and increasing your number of capillaries.

CARDIO X

[30 SECONDS] *Run in Place* (knees up)

[30 SECONDS] *Run in Place* (heels to buttocks)

[30 SECONDS] *Imaginary Jump Rope*

[30 SECONDS] *Jumping Jacks*

[45 SECONDS] *Run Lunges* – Low-impact, straight-arm or pull variety.

[5 BREATHS] *Wide-Feet Forward Hamstring Stretch* – With feet wide apart, fold forward at waist with straight or slightly bent legs. Place hands on floor or fold arms directly below head.

[5 BREATHS] *Split-Leg Forward Hamstring Stretch* – Standing with feet together, take large step forward, keeping heels aligned. Turn front foot out with arms reaching skyward, exhale as you lean forward and bend torso over front leg. Use yoga block if needed. Repeat on other side.

[5 BREATHS] *Standing Quad Stretch* – Balancing on one leg, reach behind with right hand and grasp right ankle. Gently pull heel toward buttocks until stretch is felt. Repeat on other leg.

THE WORKOUT This workout is designed as an addition to your standard P90X workload on those days when you want to do an extra workout, Doubles, or as a substitute if your body needs a break from more intense cardio like Plyometrics.

The Doubles plan of attack delivers some extra cardiovascular exercise to enhance performance or weight loss. Those attempting to use Cardio X for a Doubles workout should be completely injury-free and have plenty of energy to add another workout to their schedule 3 or 4 days per week.

Workout Tools: stool or chair • mat • yoga blocks • heart rate monitor • water and towel

YOGA

SUN SALUTATIONS (VINYASAS) [2 REPS]
1

_Standing tall with feet together, inhale and raise arms straight overhead. Exhale, open arms, and swan dive forward with a flat back, bending torso over legs. Look forward until the last second, then place hands on floor next to feet. Inhale and raise torso up into flat back. Hold for beat and exhale forward, placing hands on either side of feet. Gently step or jump back into plank, then down to Chaturanga. Inhale, pulling torso forward and up into Upward Dog pose. Exhale, pushing up hips and torso into Downward Dog pose. From Downward Dog, inhale, bending knees, looking between hands, and hop feet forward to hands. Keeping hands on floor, straighten legs. Keeping back and legs strong, inhale into reverse swan dive, ending with fingers skyward and with slight back bend. Perform Vinyasa.

RUNNER'S POSE
2

_Bend over with legs split in a low forward lunge, front leg bent at 90 degrees. Knee should be over the ankle and back leg straight on the ball of foot. Fingertips barely touch the floor on either side of front foot. Perform Vinyasa and repeat on opposite side.

WARRIOR ONE
3

_From Runner's Pose, raise torso straight up and reach hands and arms skyward. Back heel should be placed on floor with front of foot turned slightly out. Perform Vinyasa and repeat on opposite side.

WARRIOR TWO
4

_Identical lower-body position to Warrior One. Starting with the right side first, extend right arm forward and left arm back, while keeping torso centered over hips. Arms should be parallel to the floor. Go back to Warrior One, then Runner's Pose, then Plank. Perform Vinyasa and repeat sequence on opposite side.

REVERSE WARRIOR
5

_From Warrior Two position, arch torso back toward rear leg, gently placing back hand on straight back leg. Opposite arm, while turning palm down, reaches and extends overhead toward back wall. Go back to Warrior Two, then Warrior One, then Runner's Pose, then Plank. Perform Vinyasa and repeat sequence on opposite side.

KENPO

BALL KICK
6

[20 REPS EACH SIDE]

_Keep elbows in tight and hands up when kicking out. Be sure to rotate hips. Repeat same sequence on other side.

HOOK/UPPERCUT/ SIDE KICK
7

[15 REPS EACH SIDE]

_From Fighter's Stance with left foot forward, Hook left, Uppercut right, and Side Kick right. Repeat same sequence on other side.

FRONT & BACK KNUCKLES/ BALL KICK/BACK KICK
8

[15 REPS EACH SIDE]

_From Fighter's Stance, Knuckle Front and Back, followed by Ball Kick (front), then Back Kick. Repeat same sequence on other side.

JAB/CROSS/HOOK/UPPERCUT
9 [25 REPS EACH SIDE]

_Keep abs in tight and rotate your hips. Repeat same sequence on other side.

THREE-DIRECTION KICK
10 [18 REPS EACH SIDE]

_The form that applies to these kicks separately still applies in combination. Always lean in opposite direction of every kick. This will allow you to achieve greater kick height and avoid injury. Repeat same sequence on other side.

TO INTENSIFY: *Avoid tapping floor with foot between each kick.*

AIRBORNE HEISMAN
11 [30 SECONDS]

_This is a lateral leaping exercise. Start with feet together and jump sideways. As soon as you land, bring opposite knee to your chest. Repeat back and forth.

SWING KICK
12 [30 SECONDS]

_Stand directly behind a chair or stool and lift first one leg, then the other back and forth over the chair. Modify by keeping knees bent over back of chair and control speed.

TO INTENSIFY: *Use a stool for more height, and place hands behind head or straight up in the air.*

JUMP SHOT
13 [30 SECONDS]

_Catch with one hand and shoot with the other.

TIRE
14 [30 SECONDS]

_Similar to Airborne Heisman, but traveling 4 wide steps forward, then 4 wide steps back. No grabs or poses.

TO INTENSIFY: *Pick up speed and height.*

WACKY JACKS
15 [30 SECONDS]

_Like jumping jacks, but wacky with side crunches.

REPEAT PREVIOUS SEQUENCE

SQUAT X-PRESS
16 [30 REPS]

_Squat and extend arms up (overhead) and out to create an "X."

TO INTENSIFY: *Add jump at end of move.*

STEAM ENGINE
17 [50 REPS]

_Standing with feet shoulder-width apart, clasp hands behind head, keeping elbows wide. Alternate left elbow to right knee while focusing on keeping head and chest up. Go from side to side and increase speed every 10 reps. Each left-right combo counts as 1 rep.

DREYA ROLL
18 [60 SECONDS]

_From standing position, roll onto back. Kick legs straight up and roll forward, propelling body to a standing position. Use hands to get up.

TO INTENSIFY: *Increase speed and pace. Try without using hands. Jump at end.*

SQUAT RUN
19 [30 SECONDS EACH SIDE]

_From squat position, move arms back and forth as if running.

TO INTENSIFY: *Get lower and increase speed of arms.*

SUPERMAN/BANANA
20 [60 SECONDS]

_Lying on stomach, extend legs and arms straight out in front. Try to get as much of your body off floor as possible. Then roll to your back, keeping your legs and arms extended straight out approximately 6 to 12 inches off floor (biceps should be beside ears). Move back and forth between these positions for a 3-count hold, for a total of 1 minute. Always maintain a softball-size space between chin and chest.

TO INTENSIFY: *Increase height of arms and legs in both positions while still maintaining proper form.*

BURN, BURN, BURN.

COOL-DOWN AND STRETCH

[30 SECONDS] *Easy Run in Place with Upper-Body Ballistic Stretches*

Shakers – Shake out body.

Huggers – Swing arms as if giving yourself a hug, alternating arm position every 20 seconds.

[5 BREATHS] *Wide-Feet Forward Hamstring Stretch* – With feet wide apart, fold forward at waist with straight or slightly bent legs. Place hands on floor or fold arms directly below head.

Downward Dog with Calf Stretch – In Downward Dog position, separate feet hip-distance apart. Slowly alternate bending one knee while straightening opposite leg and driving its heel into the ground.

[2 REPS] *Cat Stretch* – On hands and knees (hands directly beneath shoulders and knees directly under hips), round back while exhaling and drop chin to chest. Reverse move, inhaling while arching back and lifting head.

[20 SECONDS EACH SIDE] *Standing Quad Stretch* – From standing position, reach left hand behind body to grasp left leg, then pull heel up towards rear until you feel the stretch. Repeat on other side.

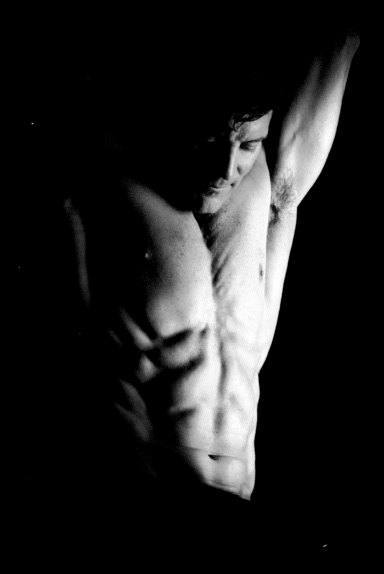

In spite of what pop culture would have us believe, showing off your six-pack is the least important reason for doing ab and core work. The muscles of your midsection are a crucial power source—it's where you transmit force between your upper and lower body. No athlete, regardless of the sport, can succeed without a solid **AB RIPPER X** core foundation. The resulting washboard is merely a bonus! The variety of movements in Ab Ripper X leaves no muscle unscathed. It's extreme work that's better than any machine in any club.

"Core training is essential to any function of daily life. Whether it be sport, getting in and out of the car, picking up your baby, getting up from your desk, or playing weekend warrior, core training incorporates all essential movement for your daily life."

—Isabelle Lorca, UCLA Strength and Functional Movement Coach

THE WORKOUT

Level 1: 15 to 20 reps   Level 2: 20 to 25 reps

All exercises are performed on the mat.

Workout Tools: mat • water and towel

IN AND OUT
1

_Sit on floor with hands at sides, knees bent, and feet on floor. Raise feet off floor and bring knees in toward your chest. Straighten legs back out and repeat movement. To increase difficulty, raise arms straight overhead.

SEATED BICYCLE
2 [50 REPS]

_Sitting in same position as In and Out, make small circles with legs as if pedaling a bicycle. Do 25 reps forward and 25 reps backward (1 revolution = 1 rep). To increase difficulty, raise arms straight overhead.

SEATED CRUNCHY FROG
3

_Sit on the floor with knees bent toward ceiling and wrap your hands around your knees. Next, extend your legs straight out to a 45-degree angle as your arms open out to your sides, level with shoulders. Fold knees back in and wrap your arms around them, keeping feet off the ground.

CROSSED LEG/WIDE LEG SIT-UP
4

_Lie flat on back with feet crossed OR legs wide. Place one hand behind head and bring torso up to perform standard sit-up movement. Reach other arm out to touch opposite foot. Alternate arm positions for each rep. If unable to keep feet planted firmly on floor, use dumbbell(s) to help anchor lower body.

FIFER SCISSOR
5

_Lie flat on your back, extending one leg skyward, while lifting opposite leg off the floor a few inches. Alternate legs in scissor motion for a 3-count hold for every rep. Keep both feet flexed throughout entire exercise.

HIP ROCK 'N' RAISE
6

_Lie on back, open hips, and bend legs so the bottoms of your feet are touching. With arms at sides, rock your hips, lift pelvis, and drive feet directly up towards ceiling (toes straight up, NOT over face). When lowering legs back down, don't let them touch the floor.

PULSE-UP (HEELS TO HEAVEN)
7

_Lying on back, extend legs straight up with arms at sides. When raising hips, imagine touching the ceiling with the balls of your feet. Be sure to lift the legs straight up at 90 degrees, and NOT at an angle toward head. Focus on maintaining straight legs.

ROLL-UP/V-UP COMBO
8

_Lie flat on back with legs straight out and arms extended straight up toward ceiling. Bring body up as if doing a standard sit-up, touching hands to toes. Slowly lower torso toward floor, while simultaneously bringing legs up off floor at 45 degrees. Bring torso back up and reach for your toes while legs are in the air. Imagine creating a jackknife position with your body. Lower entire body to starting position and repeat sequence.

OBLIQUE V-UP
9

_Lie on right side with legs at a 30-degree angle and right arm straight along torso. Place left arm behind head and lift legs and torso simultaneously, driving elbow toward knee. Keep legs and shoulders off floor once you begin. Switch sides and repeat movement.

LEG CLIMB
10

_Lie on back with one leg bent and foot flat on the floor. The other leg should be extended straight out at a 45-degree angle. Climb leg with alternating hands. Do not bend extended leg while climbing leg. Repeat sequence on other leg.

Version 1: 4 leg grabs (thigh, calf, ankle, toe)

Version 2: 2 leg grabs (calf, toe)

Version 3: Straight to toe

MASON (KAYAK) TWIST
11 [40 REPS]

_While seated, clasp hands together and raise feet 4 to 6 inches off mat. Twist upper torso from side to side, touching knuckles on each side of floor.

STRETCH

Cobra Stretch – Lie flat on stomach and raise upper body by straightening arms and pushing off floor. Keep chest up and shoulders back. Thighs should rest on the floor.

Child's Pose – Sitting on knees, fold body over legs and relax head and arms on floor.